William Nixon was Professor of Obstetrics and Gynaecology in the University of London and Director of Obstetrics at University College Hospital for twenty years. The son of a professor, he was born in Malta in 1903 and educated at Epsom College, before studying medicine at St Mary's Hospital, Paddington, which he entered as a scholar. Specializing in obstetrics, he was on the consultant staff of two London hospitals before going to Hong Kong in 1935 as University Professor in that branch of medicine. He returned to London in 1938 and, after working at the Soho Hospital for Women, became Professor of Obstetrics at Istanbul University in 1943. Professor Nixon was a member of several foreign obstetrics and gynaecological societies, and received the Petrus Pazmany Medal from Budapest University in 1947. Apart from papers in medical journals he published *A Guide to Obstetrics in General Practice* (1954). He died in 1966.

Geoffrey Chamberlain is a consultant obstetrician at a teaching hospital in London. He qualified from University College Hospital, London, in 1954, became a Fellow of the Royal College of Surgeons, a member of the Royal College of Obstetricians and Gynaecologists and was awarded an M.D. of the University of London in 1968. Mr Chamberlain has written widely in medicine and lectures extensively in the U.S.A. and Great Britain. His major research interest is Fetal Physiology and he is actively concerned with ante-natal care and counselling patients about pregnancy and childbirth. With the rapid evolution of safe scientific obstetrics, he feels that the patient may sometimes be left not understanding the reasons for many of the procedures. He is married to a doctor and they live in South London with their five children.

WILLIAM NIXON

CHILDBIRTH

**REVISED BY
GEOFFREY CHAMBERLAIN**

PENGUIN BOOKS

Penguin Books Ltd, Harmondsworth, Middlesex, England
Penguin Books Inc., 7110 Ambassador Road, Baltimore, Maryland 21207, U.S.A.
Penguin Books Australia Ltd, Ringwood, Victoria, Australia
Penguin Books Canada Ltd, 41 Steelcase Road West, Markham, Ontario, Canada
Penguin Books (N.Z.) Ltd, 182–190 Wairau Road, Auckland 10, New Zealand

First published by Gerald Duckworth, 1955
Published in Penguin Books 1961
Reprinted 1963, 1965, 1967, 1969
Second edition (revised by Geoffrey Chamberlain) 1975

Copyright © the Estate of W. C. W. Nixon, 1955
Copyright © Geoffrey Chamberlain, 1975

Made and printed in Great Britain
by C. Nicholls & Company Ltd
Set in Monotype Times

This book is sold subject to the condition
that it shall not, by way of trade or otherwise,
be lent, re-sold, hired out, or otherwise circulated
without the publisher's prior consent in any form of
binding or cover other than that in which it is
published and without a similar condition
including this condition being imposed
on the subsequent purchaser

TABLE OF CONTENTS

List of Figures	7
Preface to the Second Edition	9
1 Introduction	11
2 Diagnosis of Pregnancy	15
3 Development of the Baby	25
4 The Changing Months in Pregnancy	36
5 Ante-natal Care	44
6 Delivery of the Baby	61
7 Post-natal Care	79
8 Baby Care and Feeding	92
9 Problems in Pregnancy	101
10 Some Questions Mothers Ask	111
Glossary	121

LIST OF FIGURES

1	A vaginal examination	19
2	Growth of the fetus in early pregnancy	20
3	An obstetric calculation table	23
4	The uterus, the vagina and the Fallopian tubes	25
5	The relationship of menstruation, ovulation and the safe period	27
6	The relative sizes of a human sperm and an ovum	28
7	Division of the fertilized ovum	29
8	Microscopic structure of part of the placenta	31
9	Growth of the uterus in pregnancy	32
10	Rate of growth of the fetus and the newborn baby	33
11	Size of the uterus at the three stages of pregnancy	38
12	The pressure of the growing fetus on the underside of the diaphragm	42
13	The spacing of ante-natal visits	48
14	The cervix in labour	64
15	The stages in labour	68
16	The pelvic diaphragm	122
17	Lie of the fetus	123
18	Presentation of the fetus	125

PREFACE TO THE REVISED EDITION

CHILDBIRTH is written mainly for pregnant women, but also for fathers, midwives in training and the many people who now want to know the facts about pregnancy and childbirth. The days when events of reproduction were shrouded in mystery are over and in this decade there are many facilities for the mother to find out what is happening to her and to her unborn child. Ante-natal instruction classes are widespread and many pamphlets and books deal with aspects of having a baby. Doctors and midwives are much more ready to answer questions, but many women find it difficult to phrase these questions. The authors of this book – consultant obstetricians who span a professional lifetime of forty years – have based this book on the questions asked by many thousands of women. It is hoped that reading it will answer many questions as yet unasked and that it will stimulate further inquiries which can be taken up with the woman's own medical advisers.

Professor William Nixon, the original author of this book, died in February 1966. He had been a teacher of the University of London at University College Hospital. It was not only doctors and midwives, however, whom Will Nixon taught; he was one of the first men to be aware of the need of teaching the mothers themselves, and many who were cared for at U.C.H. in the 1940s and 1950s bear testimony to this. He started a series of instructional classes for mothers and their husbands so that they approached the events of labour forearmed. He was one of the most experienced in the field of ante-natal education and the book *Childbirth* was one of the results of this. A man of great integrity and kindness, he knew his patients, his midwives and his fellow doctors as individuals.

The present author was one of Professor Nixon's pupils and from him learnt the beginnings of his obstetrics. Although now some years away from this teaching, my knowledge and attitudes to the subject have been influenced by my senior and I am pleased to try to carry on in the tradition that he started. Writing a short book like this inevitably involves leaving out a lot of things and condensing much material. There are points where others hold different opinions and would suggest different treatments, but the views expressed here are based on work in the field by Professor Nixon and myself.

On behalf of both of us, I would like to thank Dr Stuart Campbell of Queen Charlotte's Hospital for the illustration of Ultrasound, and others who lent material for illustrations. I am glad to acknowledge the helpful comments of Mrs Nina Taylor-Thomas, Superintendent Physiotherapist at Queen Charlotte's Hospital, who has been of great help throughout the book and particularly in those sections dealing with her subject. I would also like to thank Mrs Carol Nation who has patiently assembled and typed the repeated drafts that a book like this requires. Finally, I am appreciative of the many patients who helped by asking questions, raising points and reading the script at various stages. That their assistance was so readily given made the writing more pleasurable.

Malta 1974　　　　　　　　　　　GEOFFREY CHAMBERLAIN

Chapter 1

INTRODUCTION

NOT so very long ago it was thought to be improper to talk about pregnancy. Women were expected either to conceal the fact that a baby was on the way, or else to withdraw from the community. They were driven to seek advice from those who were not really fitted to give it. There were no midwives or doctors interested in obstetrics and maternity care rested in the hands of women like Sarah Gamp, whom Charles Dickens described so vividly in *Martin Chuzzlewit*. It was the Gamps who gave the advice and actually supervised confinements. All that has changed – the Gamps have gone and in their place we have well-trained teams of midwives and doctors.

Attitudes to pregnant women have also changed. There is a more open approach to pregnancy and childbirth, and the emotional stresses in a mother are recognized. All those who work in the field of obstetrics realize that for some women having a baby is an anxious event. A lot of this is anxiety about the unknown: it is always worse when one is uncertain and has no knowledge of what is to come. Pregnancy may be a reminder of the first visit to the dentist – far worse before you went than after you had been and knew what it was all about.

For this reason we consider that mothers should know more about pregnancy and childbirth. Pregnancy is part of everyday life, it can be fascinating and exciting. Forewarning the mother about what may happen is forearming her to deal with situations as they occur. Some of the anxieties women have at this time are attributed to the stresses of modern life. It is claimed that we should return to natural childbirth so that the mother can participate in what is a natural event – the reproduction of our species. This is an excellent thought, but in certain cases we have interfered with Nature already. For instance, we wash our hands before delivering a baby and we give drugs to stop the uterus from bleeding too much after delivery. Thus we are improving on natural events for Nature is wasteful and in Nature many mothers are permanently maimed and their offspring die. Specialists in childbirth try to prevent the worst aspects of Nature and it is a question within the judgement of your own obstetrician and midwife where the line comes between the natural and the assisted event. It is clear that, rather than return to the good old days of infection and unskilled ignorant midwifery, there is a balance to be drawn between the two extreme points of view.

There is an enormous folklore of legend and myth surrounding childbirth. Giving birth is one of the basic events of life and women from a very early age are conditioned by the tribal memory about what may happen. Much of this folklore, like other myths, is quite fictitious and bears little relation to truth, having been blown up from some smaller event several generations before. Mothers, especially those having their first baby, are told all sorts of stories about childbirth by their relations and friends. This is marketplace talk and it is not useful; the advice to listen to on childbirth is that of your doctor, midwife or health visitor.

There are three important questions that nearly all women ask themselves or their medical advisers throughout pregnancy and they often place these questions in this order:

Will my child be normal?

Will I have a normal delivery?

Will it hurt?

These three questions will be dealt with in detail in this book, for they are the basic thoughts of many pregnant women. Because they ask themselves these points and think about them, women in pregnancy quite often dream about them. Dreams are only reflections of our own innermost thoughts and there is nothing abnormal in either thinking about or subconsciously considering such situations, for everyone does. Many women go through pregnancy worrying about the fact that they are worrying, but both the basic thoughts and the dreams which follow are perfectly normal behaviour.

While with her rational mind the mother may accept what doctors and midwives tell her and she may believe all she reads in this book, there may still be lurking at the back of her mind some doubt that she may be one of the few who will be unlucky in the outcome of her pregnancy. There are women who consider that they have been unlucky all their lives – why should their luck change with pregnancy? These are the mothers who are especially overjoyed when they find they can produce a baby quite normally. Suddenly their lives change and they develop a confidence which they have never known before. Their greatest wonder is that from them has come this life – they have made a new individual.

There are certain times in pregnancy when the discomfort increases and having a baby becomes a drag. Many women take this for granted and do nothing about it. The last few weeks are perhaps the most trying times when there may be the discomfort of pressure of the baby on the stomach and backache, and, worst of all, a restlessness at night so that the mother cannot sleep. Now is the time, lying awake at night, that she cannot stop thinking of what is shortly going to happen and she imagines all sorts of things. If this happens she should talk to her doctor. He can prescribe perfectly safe sleeping tablets and she should take them for they do no harm when used for a short time. The good relaxers are the good sleepers. They are the people who do not toss and turn many times during the night; they do not wake up after eight hours' sleep still feeling tired and wanting another few hours of sleep. If you are not naturally a good relaxer, then let your doctor know and he will help you.

The pregnant woman should consider herself an athlete preparing for a big event. As we know from reading about the training of Olympic Games competitors, the physical and the mental must combine in order to produce the best performance; the woman preparing herself for childbirth should consider that she has similar training to do, both to assist the process of childbirth and to help regain a good figure after the baby is born. The physical training is not so arduous as the athlete's but it still exists and in parts of our book we will outline some ideas on this. The mental training is most important – if a mother has thought about, read about and discussed the pregnancy and labour with her medical and nursing attendants, she will be far better trained at the time of delivery. She will thus enjoy the event more and probably be more efficient in producing her baby.

One of the most discussed subjects at present is the relief of pain in childbirth. Because of scientific advances, there are now methods that are of great help in relieving the pain of labour. Everyone sympathizes with the demand that women should have this relief and if they need help medicines are close at hand. But a mother can do a lot to help herself beforehand by a better understanding of the birth process so that she enters labour with a knowledge of what is happening inside her body, both to herself and her baby. Further, if she has worked at a pattern of relaxation, she often finds that this provides something constructive to do other than think about the pain to come. Indeed, such a woman frequently finds that the stronger contractions in later labour are not correspondingly more painful and that she needs less of the analgesic drugs available.

Chapter 2

DIAGNOSIS OF PREGNANCY

It is sometimes difficult in the early weeks to be certain that pregnancy has started. There are some changes you may notice yourself, and others that your doctor can discover by examination.

Changes You May Notice

Changes in menstruation. Most women stop seeing their monthly periods when they become pregnant. You should note the date of the last normal period for it helps to date the pregnancy and so guide your doctor to work out when your baby may be expected. Some women do not menstruate exactly every twenty-eight days but most have a regular cycle of between twenty-one and thirty-five days to which they keep: this is taken into consideration when making calculations about the birth. When a period is overdue by more than two weeks and sexual intercourse has taken place, it is natural to suspect the possibility of pregnancy. By the time the second period is missed, other changes will be noticed which will probably confirm the pregnancy. The lack of a period does not automatically mean a woman is pregnant – it is possible to miss a period, particularly after emotional or physical shocks. Changes of climate or environment, fear of pregnancy or certain diseases can also be associated with absence of menstruation (amenorrhoea).

It must also be realized that it is possible to bleed from the vagina and still be pregnant. During the first three months of pregnancy there may be a blood loss which will be less than a normal period. When this happens it may make the calculation of the expected date of delivery of the baby uncertain, since the last normal menstrual period may not have been noted.

Another difficulty is dating the last normal period for those women who are taking oral contraceptives. About a fifth of the women now becoming pregnant have been on the pill until a few months before conception. They may not have established a regular menstrual cycle and it is therefore sometimes difficult to date their pregnancies as accurately as for women who are menstruating regularly and are not on the pill.

Changes in the breasts. Quite early in pregnancy the breasts become heavier and tender, and a tingling sensation often develops. These changes may be noticed within a few weeks of the missed menstrual period. The nipples are more prominent and later on there is a characteristic darkening of the pigmented area around the nipple – the areola. On this area small nodules develop which stand out from the skin. With the natural development of the breasts at this time, there is an increase of blood supply and veins can often be seen under the skin running in the direction of the nipple. Later it is possible to press out a secretion; this is the forerunner of the milk and it may escape from the breast, drying on the nipples. As pregnancy proceeds this fluid increases in amount and may escape spontaneously from the breast.

Nausea and vomiting. A feeling of nausea is quite common at the sixth to eighth week after the last normal menstrual period; this is commonly felt on rising from bed and is usually referred to as morning sickness, though it can occur at any time of the day, some women noticing it mostly in the evening. This symptom usually passes off by the twelfth week; it varies in severity but most women are not greatly

DIAGNOSIS OF PREGNANCY

inconvenienced and are able to carry on with their daily tasks.

It is not necessary for a woman to vomit in order to be certain that she is pregnant; when it does happen it is no fault of hers that she feels like this. The exact cause of the vomiting is unknown. As well as hormonal changes in the body causing a relaxation and mild distension of the stomach, it is believed that there is an emotional or psychological aspect to vomiting at this time – women who are particularly anxious or unhappy about their pregnancy are more likely to vomit: an understanding of the changes that are taking place in one's body during early pregnancy can itself help to ease this anxiety.

Sickness does not mean that pregnancy is going to be any more problematical than average. With simple advice and treatment it can be cured. If your doctor decides to ameliorate the worst effects of the sickness, the treatment he prescribes will be safe for both you and your unborn child and will usually provide a welcome relief.

Changes in urination. The mother will notice that she has to pass urine more frequently, even in the early weeks of pregnancy. Bladder irritability at this stage (due mostly to hormone changes in the body) is perfectly natural. A little later on pressure from the growing uterus is felt in the bladder but after the first three months the increased frequency of urination usually disappears. It may return in the last few weeks of pregnancy when the baby's head returns to the pelvis and presses on the bladder.

Mucous discharge. A vaginal discharge of a watery nature may be noticed. This is due to greater activity of the mucous glands of the cervix (neck of the uterus) and increased blood supply to the genital organs: this develops even in early pregnancy. If it is excessive, then the doctor should be consulted.

All these symptoms are normal and indicate the body's reaction to pregnancy. Some women may only notice a few of them whilst in a very small number they may not occur at all despite a perfectly normal pregnancy. Other women find that certain symptoms become unbearable. In this country women do not usually visit their doctor until eight to ten weeks after the last menstrual period for they feel that they do not want to bother him, but if any woman has problems before this she should not hesitate to see him right away for he can often bring relief and help.

Changes Your Doctor May Notice

When a woman goes to her doctor with any of the above symptoms he will probably examine her to see if she is pregnant. At this early stage the growing baby is very small and the changes in the uterus are not very great. Since the uterus and the growing baby are tucked deep into the bony pelvis, it will be impossible to detect any signs of early pregnancy unless the doctor can feel the enlarging uterus accurately. This means that the doctor may need to make an internal examination. Some mothers are obviously nervous about this, but a properly conducted vaginal examination is not painful and has no effect on the growing baby. This examination also ensures that all is well in the vagina for the subsequent delivery. It is often made at the first ante-natal visit and is not usually repeated at each subsequent visit.

At this examination the doctor usually passes one or two gloved fingers into the vagina and places the other hand on the abdomen (see Figure 1). He is detecting the increase in size and bulkiness of the uterus and is using this to measure the progress of early pregnancy. He is also checking the position of the uterus and ensuring that there are no other problems in that area. Sometimes it is also possible for him

DIAGNOSIS OF PREGNANCY

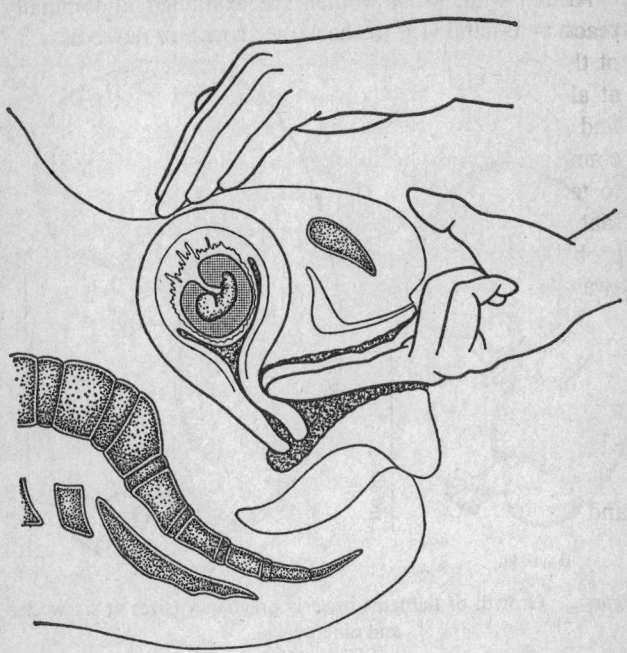

Figure 1 A vaginal examination to determine the size of the uterus.

to decide at that point whether the capacity of the pelvis is sufficient for the baby's controlled delivery. Many women build up fears about this examination, but we would stress that it is not painful in the hands of a competent doctor and is a very essential examination for the future well-being of the unborn child.

Abdominal examination. In the first twelve weeks of pregnancy the uterus has not enlarged sufficiently to be felt outside the pelvis, but after this each week is accompanied by an increase in size of the fetus (see Figure 2). This can be detected by feeling the growing uterus through the mother's abdominal wall. Most women are examined abdominally at each ante-natal visit to check the growth of the uterus.

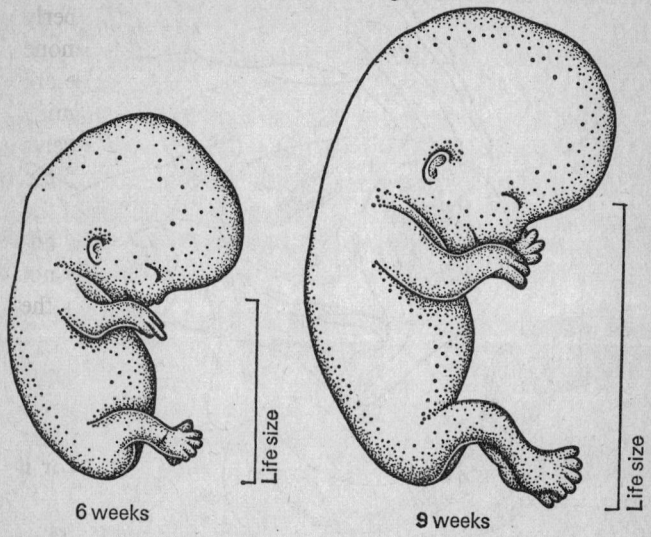

Figure 2 Growth of the fetus in early pregnancy (sizes at six weeks and nine weeks).

Fetal heart. The beats of the fetal heart are not heard with a stethoscope until the twenty-fourth week of pregnancy or even later. The doctor then places a stethoscope on the abdomen and hears the heart beating through the uterus and the mother's abdominal wall at a rate of about 140 to the minute – about twice the rate of an adult's pulse. Many obstetrical clinics now have miniature Ultrasound machines that can detect the pulsations of the fetal heart much earlier than this – from approximately twelve weeks of pregnancy.

Special pregnancy tests. There are certain tests which can be performed when there is doubt about pregnancy. They depend on examining an early morning specimen of urine for hormones but are not always absolutely reliable. When,

DIAGNOSIS OF PREGNANCY

early in pregnancy, the fertilized egg embeds itself in the wall of the uterus and grows, a hormone is developed to help growth and assist the uterus in keeping the egg properly supplied with nutrients. After use in the body, the hormone is eventually excreted and can be detected when there are adequate concentrations in the urine, thus confirming pregnancy. These tests are not used until at least twelve to fourteen days have elapsed since the first day of the missed period, i.e. five or six weeks after the first day of the last normal menstrual period. Even at this time it is advisable to repeat the test if it is negative for there may not yet be a great enough concentration of hormone in the urine.

If a test is necessary, about four ounces of the first urine passed in the day should be collected in a bottle which has been previously washed in boiled water. The specimen should be sent to a laboratory as soon as possible, for if there is excessive delay the test may prove valueless.

These tests are time-consuming and are not necessary in every pregnancy unless there is a question of urgency or of some unusual doubt. The more reliable ones will pick up 98-9 per cent of pregnancies if made at the correct time. The usual reason for failure is that the urine sample does not contain enough hormone to make the test positive. This could either be because pregnancy is not far enough advanced or because the specimen is not an early morning one and so not concentrated enough. The occasional falsely positive test is also a worry. This usually only happens in women who are producing large amounts of the hormone for some other reason. Women between the ages of forty and fifty have an increased secretion of hormones from the pituitary glands in an increased effort to stimulate the failing ovary into producing eggs. If there is any doubt about the validity of a pregnancy test it should always be repeated a week later and sometimes a doctor may decide to use a different method on the second occasion.

X-ray diagnosis. This is one of the certain ways of diagnosing pregnancy. The earliest time at which the baby's skeleton can be seen is sixteen to eighteen weeks if the angle at which the film is taken is correct. There is little point in trying to show a fetus before this time for the bones are not dense enough. However, because X-rays are a potential hazard to the unborn child, it is wiser to use other methods to confirm pregnancy if at all possible.

Ultrasound pictures. Most specialized obstetrical hospitals have equipment which can detect pregnancy in its very early stages by beaming short-wave sound waves into the uterus (the principle is similar to radar). These produce a very accurate result and are completely safe. However, such tests are only available in large hospitals at the moment.

Calculation of the Expected Date of Delivery

Pregnancy is usually considered to last about 280 days or 40 weeks. Doctors and midwives usually work with the week as their unit of time for the day implies too much precision whilst the month is too long a unit. Further, months are of irregular lengths (February with 28 days and January with 31), and confusion often arises between the use of calendar and lunar months.

Figure 3 An obstetric table to calculate the date a baby is due, working from the first day of the last menstrual period (NOT the missed period but the last one that came).

To calculate the expected date of delivery read along the *upper* line of any column; the delivery date will be the *lower* corresponding figure. (In a Leap year a woman whose last period was on 29 February would expect her baby on or about 6 December.) It must be remembered that the date calculated from this table is only a guide and can be up to a week out.

		1 2	3 4	5	6 7	8	9 10	11	12 13	14 15	16 17	18 19	20 21	22 23	24 25	26 27	28 29	30 31
January	October/November	1 2 8 9	3 4 10 11	5 12	6 7 13 14	8 15	9 10 16 17	11 18	12 13 19 20	14 15 21 22	16 17 23 24	18 19 25 26	20 21 27 28	22 23 29 30	24 25 31 1	26 27 2 3	28 29 4 5	30 31 6 7
February	November/December	1 2 8 9	3 4 10 11	5 12	6 7 13 14	8 15	9 10 16 17	11 18	12 13 19 20	14 15 21 22	16 17 23 24	18 19 25 26	20 21 27 28	22 23 29 30	24 25 1 2	26 27 3 4	28 5	
March	December/January	1 2 6 7	3 4 8 9	5 10	6 7 11 12	8 13	9 10 14 15	11 16	12 13 17 18	14 15 19 20	16 17 21 22	18 19 23 24	20 21 25 26	22 23 27 28	24 25 29 30	26 27 31 1	28 29 2 3	30 31 4 5
April	January/February	1 2 6 7	3 4 8 9	5 10	6 7 11 12	8 13	9 10 14 15	11 16	12 13 17 18	14 15 19 20	16 17 21 22	18 19 23 24	20 21 25 26	22 23 27 28	24 25 29 30	26 27 31 1	28 29 2 3	30 4
May	February/March	1 2 5 6	3 4 7 8	5 9	6 7 10 11	8 12	9 10 13 14	11 15	12 13 16 17	14 15 18 19	16 17 20 21	18 19 22 23	20 21 24 25	22 23 26 27	24 25 28 1	26 27 2 3	28 29 4 5	30 31 6 7
June	March/April	1 2 8 9	3 4 10 11	5 12	6 7 13 14	8 15	9 10 16 17	11 18	12 13 19 20	14 15 21 22	16 17 23 24	18 19 25 26	20 21 27 28	22 23 29 30	24 25 31 1	26 27 2 3	28 29 4 5	30 6
July	April/May	1 2 7 8	3 4 9 10	5 11	6 7 12 13	8 14	9 10 15 16	11 17	12 13 18 19	14 15 20 21	16 17 22 23	18 19 24 25	20 21 26 27	22 23 28 29	24 25 30 1	26 27 2 3	28 29 4 5	30 31 6 7
August	May/June	1 2 8 9	3 4 10 11	5 12	6 7 13 14	8 15	9 10 16 17	11 18	12 13 19 20	14 15 21 22	16 17 23 24	18 19 25 26	20 21 27 28	22 23 29 30	24 25 31 1	26 27 2 3	28 29 4 5	30 31 6 7
September	June/July	1 2 8 9	3 4 10 11	5 12	6 7 13 14	8 15	9 10 16 17	11 18	12 13 19 20	14 15 21 22	16 17 23 24	18 19 25 26	20 21 27 28	22 23 29 30	24 25 1 2	26 27 3 4	28 29 5 6	30 7
October	July/August	1 2 8 9	3 4 10 11	5 12	6 7 13 14	8 15	9 10 16 17	11 18	12 13 19 20	14 15 21 22	16 17 23 24	18 19 25 26	20 21 27 28	22 23 29 30	24 25 31 1	26 27 2 3	28 29 4 5	30 31 6 7
November	August/September	1 2 8 9	3 4 10 11	5 12	6 7 13 14	8 15	9 10 16 17	11 18	12 13 19 20	14 15 21 22	16 17 23 24	18 19 25 26	20 21 27 28	22 23 29 30	24 25 31 1	26 27 2 3	28 29 4 5	30 6
December	September/October	1 2 7 8	3 4 9 10	5 11	6 7 12 13	8 14	9 10 15 16	11 17	12 13 18 19	14 15 20 21	16 17 22 23	18 19 24 25	20 21 26 27	22 23 28 29	24 25 30 1	26 27 2 3	28 29 4 5	30 31 6 7

The date of delivery is calculated from the first day of the last menstrual period. One could add 280 days to this but this would be cumbersome and in practice it is easier to add one year and seven days and then deduct three months. For example, if the last period was 22 October 1974 then the expected date of delivery would be 29 July 1975. The easiest method of all is to look up the dates in an obstetrical calendar, as shown in Figure 3.

Since the actual date of fertilization is usually not known, there is often slight uncertainty when calculating the expected date of delivery. It is a mistake to think that labour will necessarily start exactly at the estimated time. It has been found that about one in ten pregnancies could go up to ten days over this time and a similar number end in the week before it. When menstruation is regular and occurs every twenty-eight days, this method of estimation is reasonably accurate, but even so not absolutely reliable.

It is important to realize that there is no completely reliable method of calculating the expected date of delivery, and you must not be disappointed if you find that you have not started your labour exactly on the estimated date. When menstruation is irregular and women are uncertain about their dates, it is very difficult to know when delivery is due. It is useful if an internal examination has been carried out early in pregnancy, for the doctor may be able to calculate the date of delivery by noting the size of the uterus at this time. This is one of the many reasons why the mother should come under the care of a doctor early in pregnancy. Should there be any further medical reasons for estimating the delivery date more accurately, then X-rays or Ultrasound will undoubtedly be used.

Chapter 3

DEVELOPMENT OF THE BABY

BEFORE describing what is taking place in the uterus during pregnancy, it will be helpful to consider the purpose of menstruation and the relation of ovulation (the production of the egg) and fertilization.

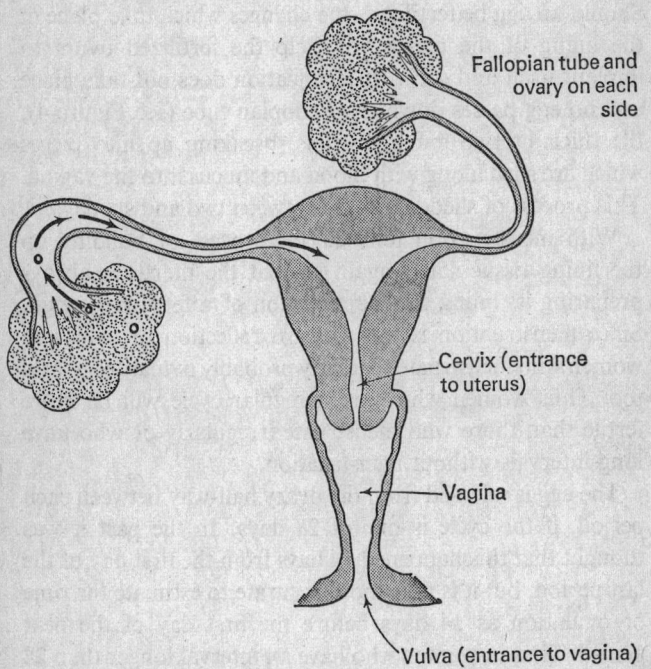

Figure 4 The uterus, the vagina and the Fallopian tubes. The inset shows the egg bursting into the Fallopian tube.

Menstruation and ovulation. Menstruation usually starts between twelve and fourteen years of age and stops between forty-five and fifty, thus delimiting the childbearing years of a woman's life. During the menstrual cycle changes take place in the lining of the uterus which are under the influence of the endocrine glands, principally the pituitary gland in the brain and the ovary in the pelvis.

Menstruation is the monthly loss of blood from the cavity of the uterus. From the day that menstruation ceases there is a gradual building up of the lining of the uterus as a suitable medium in which the fertilized egg can embed. Should an egg be fertilized, the changes which take place in the lining of the uterus will help the fertilized ovum to implant itself and grow. If fertilization does not take place and no egg passes down the Fallopian tube (see Figure 4), the thick uterine lining disrupts, breaking up into pieces which are shed along with blood and mucus into the vagina. This process of shedding takes between two and six days.

With menstruation finished, the process of building up the lining tissue starts again so that the uterus is always preparing its lining for the reception of a fertilized ovum. Since menstruation is the outward reflection of ovulation women who menstruate regularly probably ovulate regularly too. Thus women who have a regular cycle will be more fertile than those who menstruate irregularly or who have long intervals without menstruation.

The egg is released from the ovary half-way between each period, if the cycle is one of 28 days. In the past it was thought that this happened 14 days from the first day of the last period, but it is now more accurate to estimate the time of ovulation as 14 days before the first day of the next period. Thus in women who have an interval longer than 28 days, for instance 30 to 35, the date of ovulation will be later than the fourteenth day (see Figure 5). This know-

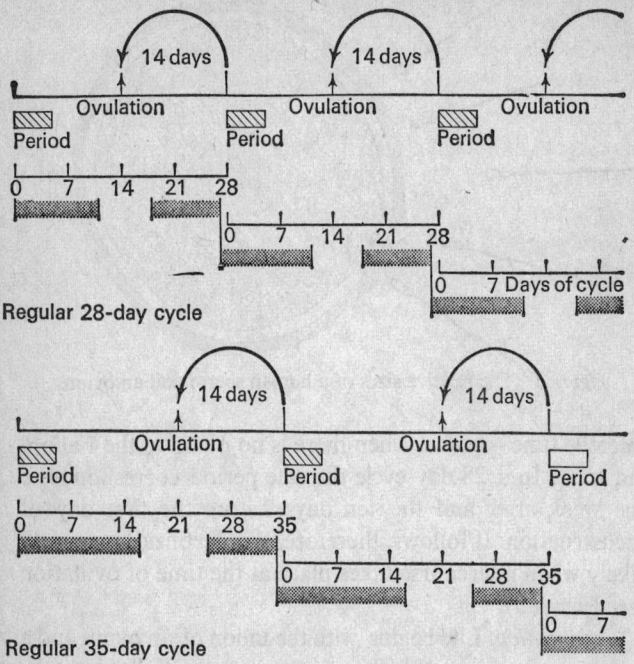

Figure 5 The relationship of menstruation, ovulation and the safe period.

ledge is important when advising about the fertile period in the cycle and also when calculating the expected date of delivery from the first day of the last period. The delivery date will be later with a longer cycle since ovulation occurs later and therefore the interval between this and the last period will be longer.

The ovum is hard to see with the naked eye, being about a quarter the size of this full-stop. It is shed from the ovary into the Fallopian tube (see Figure 4) and lives for only a few hours. This is the fertile time for it is only now that a woman becomes pregnant, whereas the safe period – the

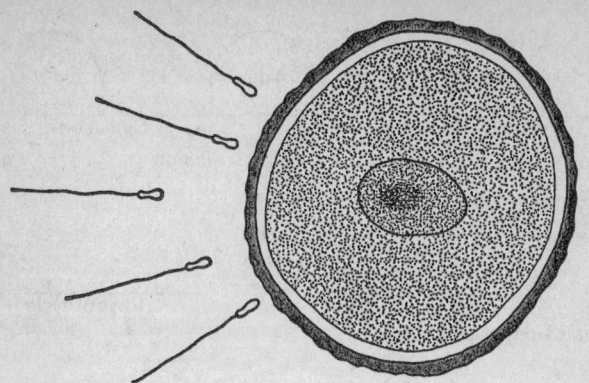

Figure 6 The relative sizes of a human sperm and an ovum.

infertile time – occurs when there is no ovum in the Fallopian tube. In a 28-day cycle the safe period corresponds to the week after and the ten days before the first day of menstruation. It follows, therefore, that fertilization is most likely when intercourse takes place at the time of ovulation (see Figure 5).

Fertilization. Life begins with the union of an ovum and a sperm (male germ cell); the ovum enters the Fallopian tube after it has been shed from the ovary. As you can see in Figure 4 the outer end of the Fallopian tube has a series of finger-like processes around it, rather like the fronds which surround the mouth of a sea anemone. These embrace the ovary just before the time of ovulation, so that when the egg is expelled from the ovary it slips straight into the Fallopian tube. It is in the outer third of this tube that fertilization takes place, not in the uterus or in the vagina as many people think.

The sperm is very much smaller than the ovum (see Figure 6) and can only be seen under a microscope. It lives for about twenty-four hours, although cases have been reported of active sperms being found as long as six days after inter-

DEVELOPMENT OF THE BABY

course. With each ejaculation up to 200 million sperms are released into the upper vagina. These move very quickly in all directions, driven by their wildly beating tails, and a large number pass upwards and enter the uterus. They negotiate the cervical canal, which is often occupied with a plug of mucus, and pass up in the fluid lining the uterus. Some reach the inner end of the Fallopian tube and a few of these will travel along its full length. Of the 200 million that started the journey perhaps only 50 or 100 sperms will finally reach the area in which an ovum is lying. Only one sperm is required to fuse with the ovum for the creation of a new life. Usually once a sperm has joined with the egg it is impossible for any of the other sperms to penetrate the egg's outer layers.

After fertilization the ovum divides and re-divides as it passes down the Fallopian tube. During these divisions this clump of cells (see Figure 7) enlarges while journeying down the tube to the uterus, taking about five days for passage. During this time the lining of the uterus is changing in preparation for the reception of the ovum; when the fertilized ovum reaches the uterine cavity, it adheres to the

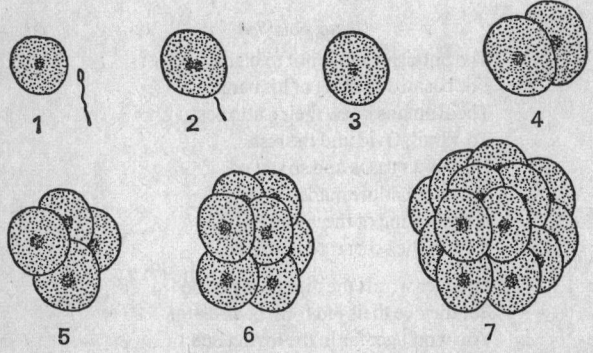

Figure 7 Division of the fertilized ovum.

wall and, by a process of erosion, embeds itself in the lining. This is a very important stage of development because if the ovum does not get a firm anchorage, an abortion or miscarriage may follow.

The embryo or fetus. It is usual to describe the conceptus up to the age of three months as an embryo and after that period of time as a fetus.

It may be confusing that this last word is spelt in two different ways; the Victorians continued the custom of spelling the word with the diphthong, foetus, but it is now realized that the more classical spelling was probably without the 'o'. If the word came from the Latin verb *feo*, then the noun fetus must be spelt with an 'e'. It is probable that the diphthong crept in during the seventh century when many other similar words were altered (e.g. *felix* – the cat – became *foelix*). There is no rationale to the spelling of many English words but at least they have some relation to their classical origin and the dropping of the 'oe' is not related to any Americanization of the language. The word can still be found spelt in either way in English books. Perhaps the situation may be made clearer by this poem about the spelling of fetus which appeared in the *Lancet* a year or two ago:

Fetus Falsified

The unborn child is not to blame
For bastard spelling of his name.
The Romans knew their Latin best.
To Virgil, Ovid and the rest
He was a FETUS and so stayed
Till later Isidore made
A diphthong of the vowel E
And so the FOETUS came to be.

To other words the diphthong came
But they've their old form back again.
You won't get far in the loving line
To tell your bird she's Foeminine.

> To call the FETUS transatlantic
> Will drive the learned men quite frantic.
> Ere Norsemen on Cape Cod were wrecked,
> The spelling FETUS was correct.

The placenta. The placenta starts to develop at the time of the embedding of the ovum. It is rather like a dinner plate in size at the end of pregnancy – about nine inches in diameter, and one inch thick. It is called the afterbirth since it is delivered after the baby, but its real importance is during pregnancy when it acts as an exchange station between the mother and her unborn baby (see Figure 8). It consists of masses of finger-like processes containing minute blood vessels which embed in the lining of the uterus. The vessels join together as they run towards the umbilical cord connecting the fetus to the placenta. Through the large vessels of

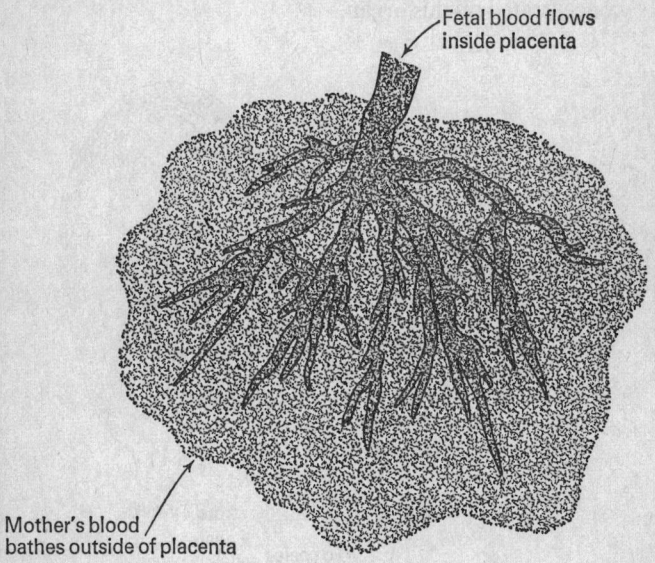

Figure 8 Microscopic structure of part of the placenta.

the umbilical cord, fetal blood is carried to the placenta and back to the fetus. The mother's blood does not mix with that of the fetus since the two circulations are separated by a membrane. In the finger-like processes of the placenta, diffusion of vital food substances and oxygen occurs from the mother's blood to that of the fetus and in return waste products from the fetus pass into the mother's circulation (see Figure 8). It will be appreciated that the placental exchange is of great importance to the fetus. Fetal life is dependent on it – if the placenta is dislodged the fetus is jeopardized. Fortunately some of the finger-like processes provide an excellent anchor, making a bond with the uterine wall. Fetal well-being in pregnancy is dependent upon the normal functioning of the placenta; in the last few years we have been learning more as much scientific research is being concentrated on this organ.

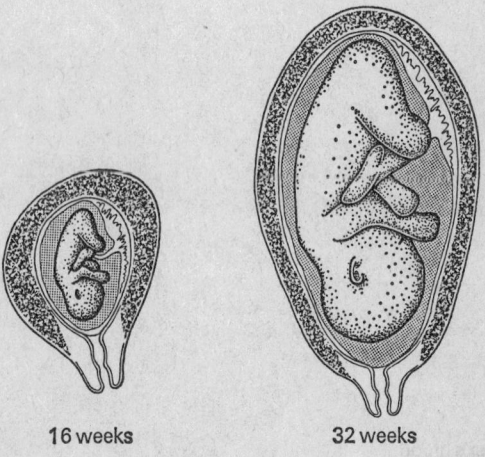

16 weeks   32 weeks

To scale

Figure 9 Growth of the uterus in pregnancy.

DEVELOPMENT OF THE BABY

The growing embryo. As the embryo grows, changes take place in the containing bag of membranes attached all round the edge of the placenta. This sac encloses an increasing amount of fluid so that the future baby's development occurs in a fluid environment. Outside all these structures are the walls of the uterus which stretch as the baby grows (see Figure 9). The fluid is a buffer preventing the fetus from injury caused by sudden jars or jolts or even direct injury to the mother's abdomen. It insulates the fetus, maintaining an even temperature, allows the limbs to move freely, and provides a comfortable medium in which to live.

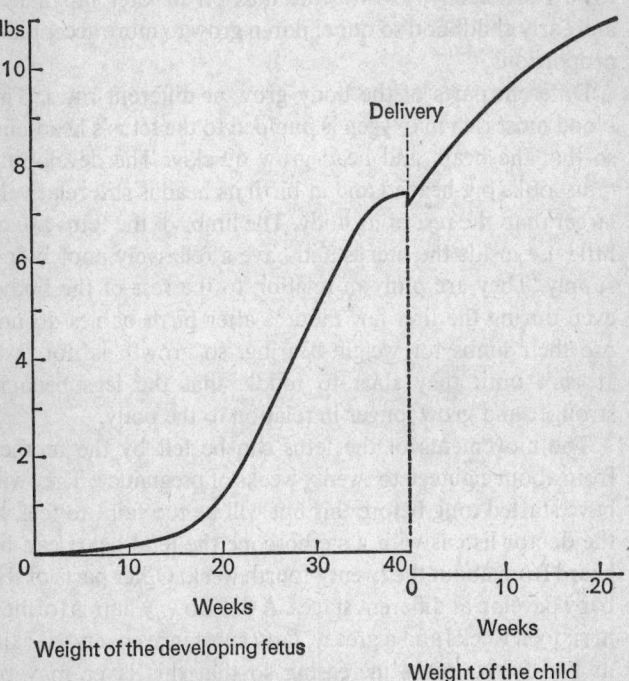

Figure 10 Rate of growth of the fetus and the newborn baby.

By the end of pregnancy, the amount of this clear fluid varies from one to four pints. It has to come away at the time of labour – one of the ways that labour starts is by bursting the 'waters' in this bag.

The fetus grows very rapidly inside the uterus. During the first nine weeks all the organs in the body are differentiating and developing. After this time, the fetus is complete and any further development is by growth. This is the time of fastest growth-rate in the whole of one's lifetime (see Figure 10). If it were continued in later life, by fifteen years of age the child would be seventy-five feet tall and weigh several tons. Fortunately, growth-rate tails off in later pregnancy and early childhood so our children grow to more acceptable proportions.

Different parts of the body grow at different rates. The blood most rich in oxygen is pumped to the fetus's head-end so that the brain and head grow quickly. The developing fetus looks big-headed and at birth its head is still relatively larger than the rest of its body. The limbs of the fetus are of little use inside the uterus and have a relatively poor blood supply. They are puny in relation to the rest of the body; even during the first few months after birth babies do not use their limbs for weight-bearing, so growth is not fast. It isn't until they start to toddle that the legs become stronger and grow longer in relation to the body.

The movements of the fetus can be felt by the mother from about eighteen to twenty weeks of pregnancy. They will have started long before this but will be too faint to feel. If the doctor listens with a stethoscope the fetal heart can be heard from about the twenty-fourth week. Other parts of the baby develop at different stages. A fine downy hair is formed at sixteen weeks and a greasy, fatty substance covers the skin at twenty-six weeks increasing so that this layer may be quite thick by birth. This fatty coating acts as an external

DEVELOPMENT OF THE BABY

protection to the baby, for most of the fat in the tissues under the baby's skin is not deposited until th last four weeks of pregnancy. This is why a baby born prematurely has a wrinkled skin and looks so wizened.

The usual weight of a full-term normal baby is 7–7½ lb. (3–3.5 kg.), with boys weighing a little more than girls. Its length is about 20 inches (50 centimetres) and, again, boys are often a little longer. A baby who is underweight at birth is not necessarily abnormal or premature. There are many reasons for the weight not being up to average and perfectly healthy babies can be born at the calculated date and yet be under the normal weight. For purposes of statistics, it is internationally agreed that a baby weighing 5½ lb. (2.5 kg.) or less should be classified as premature.

The body of the newborn baby is, of course, not the mirror image of the adult. As well as the head being large in proportion to the trunk, the legs are bent, sometimes quite acutely, at the knee and ankle joints, but they will straighten with growth. The skin is usually pink and the amount of hair varies. Some babies are born with a mass of hair, others with a scanty growth and sometimes the hair takes months to grow. It is usually dark in colour at birth but it does not always remain so; if family hair colours are lighter, it will often change in the subsequent months. The nails are normal and extend just beyond the finger-tips. The colour of the eyes often changes as the baby gets older and his eyes often do not react to light to begin with.

Chapter 4

THE CHANGING MONTHS IN PREGNANCY

The First Three Months

ONE or more periods may have been missed before pregnancy is diagnosed. The physical changes are not pronounced at first but increase during this time. Those in the breasts are probably the most noticeable for the enlargement of the uterus is not perceived by the mother at this stage. A slight watery mucous discharge from the vagina is quite normal and is due to the activity of the glands in the neck of the uterus (cervix). The urge to pass water more frequently is due to hormone changes in the body affecting the bladder muscle but the sensation is made worse by pressure of the growing uterus on the bladder; this usually diminishes after the twelfth week. Sometimes there is irritation in the vagina which should be investigated if it is excessive or persists. Normal sexual relations are often stopped voluntarily during the first few months in case intercourse should disturb the pregnancy and so lead to a miscarriage. A normally implanted embryo is extremely unlikely to be affected by sexual relations and after the first few weeks have passed there is no reason why normal activities should not be resumed. Should there be any spotting of blood from the vagina, however, it would be wise to avoid intercourse until advice has been taken from a doctor.

The emotional changes at this stage may be marked and show themselves in a variety of ways. There is a feeling of being 'different' which some women seem to notice early in pregnancy. They find themselves unable to concentrate and perhaps already have a distaste for certain foods. They may even have a feeling of dizziness and faintness once the diagnosis of pregnancy is considered. Some women become depressed and sad or even bad-tempered while others are elated and overjoyed at the prospect of having a baby. There are certain aversions and cravings which are very difficult to explain. Some foods may be found distasteful and a heavy smoker may find that she develops a loathing for cigarettes or the smell of tobacco around her. Sometimes these cravings can be for unobtainable articles or foods which are out of season, such as shrimps or exotic fruits. The importance of diet will be discussed later, but at this point it is advisable to try to resist the attempt to satisfy these more abnormal cravings. This applies especially when there is such an acute appetite and feeling of hollowness in the stomach which can only be controlled by eating enormous quantities of bulky food such as chunks of bread, several jam tarts, large numbers of pastries or lots of sweets. Some women have been told that they must feed for two when they become pregnant but this is wrong: you must control your appetite throughout the whole of pregnancy, no matter how hungry you are.

The Middle Three Months

By this time the feeling of nausea or actual sickness will have passed and many women will now feel happier and more at ease with their pregnancy. The physical changes associated with the growing fetus soon become more evident. Distension of the lower abdomen will be noticed, particularly at about the fourteenth to sixteenth week. Figure 11 shows the approximate size of the uterus according to the stage of pregnancy. There is a fullness of the abdominal wall which is noticed by the mother. She often feels selfconscious about it but other people will not see this change until several weeks after she has become aware of it. The stomach does not stick forward at this stage and often, if the muscles are good, obvious stomach enlargement does not show until twenty to twenty-four weeks of pregnancy.

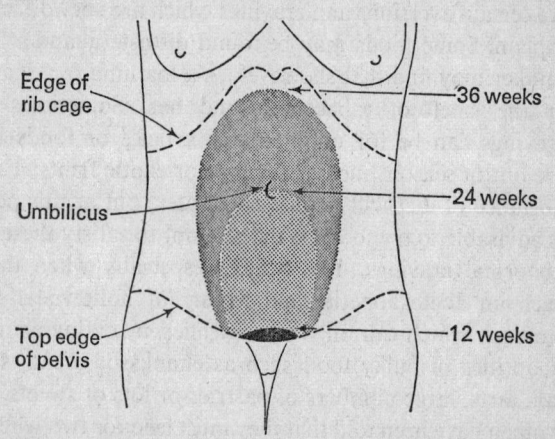

Figure 11 Size of the uterus at the three stages of pregnancy.

From some time after the eighteenth week of pregnancy the mother will feel the movements of the fetus, known as 'quickening'. In the first pregnancy it may be some time before she appreciates these gentle movements which resemble a tapping, fluttering or flickering within the uterus. Once noticed the sensation is never forgotten in subsequent pregnancies, and in consequence is often noticed then even earlier than the eighteenth week. It is advisable to make a note of the time when these movements are first felt for this information can be helpful confirmatory evidence when calculating the date of delivery.

From the earlier weeks of pregnancy, weight will start to increase. This is due not only to the growing baby and the growth of the breasts and uterus but also to the increase of fat on the shoulders, arms, thighs and legs. It should be stressed again that it is important to control weight gain during pregnancy.

A darkening of the skin or pigmentation may be noticed on the upper part of the cheeks and forehead (the 'mask of pregnancy'). This change also occurs on the nipple areas or areolae of the breasts which go from pink to brown; this is more noticeable in light-skinned women than those with darker skins and is usually a permanent change. In some women a further line of pigmentation appears vertically in the skin of the abdomen from the umbilicus down to the pubis; this is more usual in dark-skinned women. With the stretching of the abdominal wall, little stretch scars may be seen just under the skin. These short pale marks may also be found on the buttocks, thighs and breasts. There is nothing very much that you can do about these although some women do find it helpful to rub the skin with a good quality lanolin or a moisturizing cream. Although these may not disappear completely after pregnancy, their size and colour will lessen after the baby is born.

At this stage most women feel very well and often want to do a lot more than in earlier pregnancy. Having passed the first few months, the body is used to the pregnancy and many women now feel in better health. They try to extend their activities, often by great plans of home redecoration in readiness for the new baby. It must be appreciated, however, that there is an alteration in the distribution of blood around the body with more blood going to the pelvis and so relatively less to the muscles of the legs, the back and to other organs. In consequence the mother will feel tired; this is a normal accompaniment of pregnancy. If you were carrying around a heavy suitcase you would occasionally pause and put it down in order to have a rest. The burden of pregnancy cannot be put down but the changes described are going on and it is advisable for the mother to rest from time to time. Even though she is feeling perfectly well, an hour's rest on a bed every afternoon in later pregnancy is a good idea for it prevents tiredness and will help her get through the rest of the day reasonably unfatigued. This rest cannot be taken to the same extent in an armchair or on a sofa. It should be under the bedcovers and with the outer clothes removed. By all means take a book, a wireless or even the television set into the bedroom for you do not have to sleep but you should have an hour lying down.

During these middle months you will feel that you can move quite freely, although the baby is growing all the time and the abdomen is getting bigger. Correct posture is important at this stage. Shoes with very high heels should be avoided since they throw the weight of the body forward and therefore increase the hollow of the back and so strain the muscles. One of the most common causes of backache in pregnancy is wearing high heels – they should not be more than $1\frac{1}{2}$ inches in height. As pregnancy advances there is more weight in front of you and your back muscles have to adjust to this alteration. With the tilting of the pelvis you have to learn to stand so as to lessen the strain on these muscles. By standing and walking correctly you will find that the increased bulk you have to carry is not too much of an undue burden.

The Last Three Months

The main change noticed now is the increase in size of the abdomen. The movements and increased size of the baby on the stomach may cause some indigestion and heartburn. At this time the mother's movements will not be so easy and, quite naturally, there will be some breathlessness on exer-

THE CHANGING MONTHS IN PREGNANCY

tion. It will sometimes be difficult for her to get comfortable when sitting in a chair and particularly at night when lying in bed but by placing pillows under the shoulders or in the small of the back she can eventually find an acceptable position.

The pressure of the baby in the uterus and the kicking of his legs will sometimes cause a feeling of soreness under the ribs. It is this pressure also which will give a feeling of fullness in the pit of the stomach and may also produce indigestion after meals. The mother can avoid this feeling by sitting up as much as possible with the back straight; the indigestion can be relieved by having small, frequent meals.

As pregnancy approaches its end there is often a return of increased frequency in passing urine. The baby's head enters the pelvis in the last few weeks by engagement and so presses on the bladder. This irritates the bladder, allowing less urine to be stored so that urination is frequent. At this stage there may also be some weakness in the supports to the bladder so that a drop or two of urine will escape on sneezing or coughing. This is a normal event and full control will be restored after the baby is born.

During the last few weeks of pregnancy there may be an associated relief of pressure in the upper stomach for the whole baby moves down when the head engages in the pelvis (see Figure 12). Sometimes less movement of the baby is noticed and mothers become anxious thinking that all is not as it should be. There is no known explanation for the baby's activity and why he is more active at certain times than at others. His movements bear little relation to his well-being – a temporary lack of them is nothing to worry about.

If you are not sleeping during the last few weeks tell your doctor. He can prescribe mild, safe treatments to help you sleep normally. It is important to go to your doctor for he

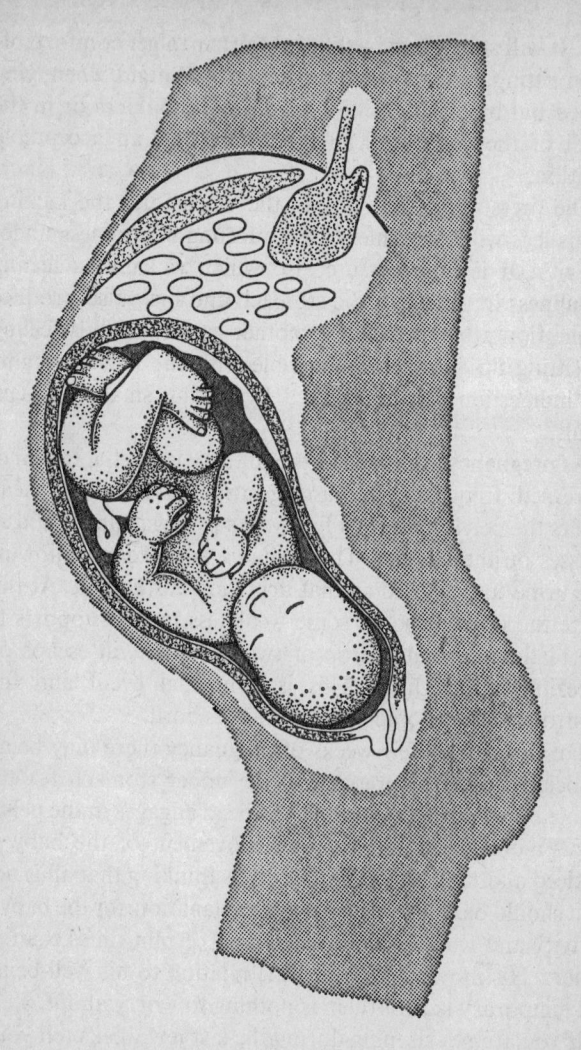

Figure 12 The pressure of the growing fetus on the underside of the diaphragm, pushing up all the intestines and the stomach into a space about a third of that they normally occupy. The upper stomach is thus often pushed up alongside the gullet and acid stomach juice refluxes up.

knows what is safe for you and the unborn baby. A part of this sleeplessness may be due to anxiety, but if you have been properly supervised and you understand the changes taking place during pregnancy and the process of birth, you will find these worries become a lot less if you get a good night's sleep.

There may be some swelling of the ankles at this time. This may simply be due to increasing pressure caused by the growing uterus, but you should always draw the attention of your medical attendant to its presence. There may also be some swelling of the fingers. Again, this should be mentioned to your doctor, who will advise you about it.

Chapter 5

ANTE-NATAL CARE

THE main purposes of ante-natal care are to supervise the health of the expectant mother and to protect her and her unborn baby from complications. The aim is to produce a healthy mother and baby who are both unscathed by pregnancy and the process of childbirth. An important part of this is the proper instruction of the mother so that she knows what is happening in pregnancy and to give her confidence for what will occur in labour. Some years ago the World Health Organization in Geneva advised that pregnant mothers should be given information about the following matters:

Physiology of pregnancy and childbirth.

Body changes and changes of mood or attitude during pregnancy.

Sexual relations during pregnancy.

Explanation of the purpose of examination procedures.

Physical and psychological preparation for labour.

Reassurance and explanation regarding unusual developments during pregnancy.

Physiological and psychological care of the infant.

All medical authorities would agree with the definitions of maternity care described above, but it is disconcerting to note that in many parts of the world millions of women have no maternity care at all. In large parts of the Third World, women go through pregnancy doing their daily tasks as best they can. When labour comes, some female relative or 'guid woman' from the village comes and helps. Under these circumstances, the loss of life and damage to both the mothers and their babies is very great. In Great Britain there have been great improvements in maternity care with the development of maternity and child welfare services during the last half century, and much ill health in the expectant mother and her baby has thus been prevented. However, many women are still not receiving the ante-natal care they might. Doctors, midwives and clinics are available and should be visited for these consultations are important to the future life and health not just of mothers but of their unborn children. Childbearing is essentially a physiological process, and the main emphasis in maternity care should be on the maintenance of a normal state. Occasionally abnormalities do occur, some of which have grave consequences but these can often be prevented or minimized by adequate pre-natal supervision.

Home or Hospital Delivery?

In the 1970s an increasing number of women are having their babies in hospital or in General Practitioner-run maternity units, and now about 85 per cent of women giving birth in England and Wales are so confined. In Scotland the proportion is very much higher. In the big towns, domiciliary deliveries are uncommon – in West London 96 per cent of babies are born in maternity units. It is probable that over the years even more women will have their babies in such places and fewer will elect to have their baby at home. There is a hangover of past years when there was a shortage of hospital beds and in some parts of the country this still applies to a limited extent. Only women having their first baby or those with some medical condition can get into hospital. In the next few years, with shorter hospital stay after delivery, it is hoped that there will soon be a maternity bed available for any woman who wants one.

It is always a wrench to leave home, particularly when there are other children in the family, and many women would like to have a domiciliary confinement for this reason. Nevertheless, it must be realized that however safe an unborn child may seem to be and however normally events may seem to be proceeding, there may be a slight risk of potential problems. Some of these cannot be foreseen and so it is wiser to have one's baby in hospital if possible. Only there are the specialist doctors who are able to help the mother or her child during childbirth. There too are the midwives trained to cover for twenty-four hours of the day, and the blood and anaesthetic services, diagnostic and pathological laboratories – all able to look after the mother and her child. These are not available in the home and although emergency cover can be obtained from the hospital in cases of domiciliary confinement, it is not as good as the hospital service itself.

It is, however, still true that the home is a more familiar and comfortable place to be, provided there are no complications. This can only be said when the delivery is over and in retrospect all can be recognized as having proceeded normally. Although obstetricians can pick out 'high risk' and 'low risk' groups, these only recognize the mathematical probabilities of a given group – no one can accurately foretell the outcome of labour for an individual woman. The times of maximum risk to both mother and baby are labour and delivery. Hence a reasonable compromise is now being reached in this country whereby women go into hospital to have their baby but return home very soon afterwards. It is the time spent in hospital after delivery that some women find irksome. In many areas of the country, a planned discharge can be made forty-eight hours after delivery and the mother can return from the care of the hospital medical and nursing staff to the family doctor and community midwife; this has to be arranged in advance. It is hoped that since the coming together of the community and hospital medical services in 1974, the artificial divisions between these two parts of the Health Service team will be reduced and then more women will come into hospital for the time of maximum need and go back to their homes very soon afterwards, having been looked after by the same doctors and midwives in both environments.

Ante-natal Visits

Ante-natal visits are spaced so that the mother sees the doctor at the correct intervals according to the need of the particular stage of pregnancy.

Most women attend for their first visit at about ten to twelve weeks. This is the longest visit and the most thorough; the mother will be asked about details of any past illnesses or operations which could be relevant to this current pregnancy. She may be asked about any illnesses in the family, such as high blood pressure or diabetes. Should she have had a baby before, this could obviously be very relevant and details of any previous pregnancies and deliveries may be required. All this information is confidential and is only asked to be of help in keeping the mother and her unborn child well during the pregnancy.

At the first visit there is very often a complete physical examination. The doctor may examine the heart, lungs, spine, abdomen and legs. This is to exclude any medical condition which might be present. The size of the uterus containing the baby will be important and this is often also checked at the first visit. Since the uterus is tucked deep in the pelvis an internal examination may be required (see p. 18).

At the first visit the mother may well see one of the medical social workers if she has any problems connected with the family or with her work. Arrangements can be made for her and her husband to attend ante-natal classes where they can learn more about pregnancy and the subsequent birth.

Other visits are usually at monthly intervals in early pregnancy. The doctor or midwife will take the blood pressure and examine the urine to exclude some of the problems mentioned later on and will often check the growth of the baby in the uterus by examining the abdomen. The mother will be weighed at these visits and the amount of weight gained between each visit noted. As pregnancy comes towards its end the visits are more frequent, becoming fortnightly and, in the last month, weekly (see Figure 13). In these later visits, the lie of the baby (that is the way he is presenting in relation to the mother's pelvis) and his fit into the pelvis are both checked by examination through the abdominal wall.

As early as possible in pregnancy a sample of blood is

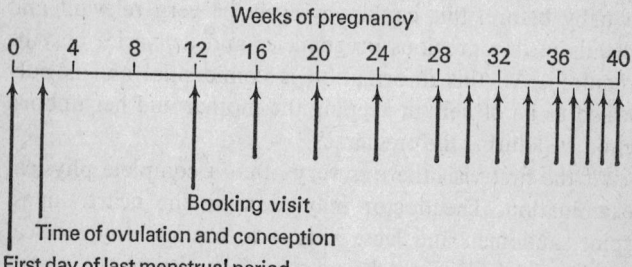

Figure 13 Example of the spacing of ante-natal visits becoming more frequent as pregnancy progresses.

ANTE-NATAL CARE

taken for blood grouping, for testing the Rhesus factor (see p. 105) and for a haemoglobin estimation. This last test checks if the mother is anaemic and may be repeated at various times during pregnancy. It is now known that by taking iron tablets during pregnancy and for a few weeks after delivery it is possible to maintain the haemoglobin in most patients at a normal level and so prevent anaemia. Further, stores of iron are built up in the mother and the baby for use in the days immediately after the birth.

A dental examination should be carried out early in pregnancy. Some clinics provide dental services, but there is no need to leave your own dentist. It used to be said that the expectant mother lost a tooth for every child. This is quite unnecessary if dental care is used properly but during pregnancy there is a tendency for fillings to loosen and gums to become sore. Your dentist can help prevent this if you consult him.

In some clinics it is still a routine to arrange for an X-ray of the lungs. By this method tuberculosis and other chest conditions can be detected and treated. Any X-ray department which takes such films will also be aware of the problems of X-rays in pregnancy and will take proper precautions to prevent any risks to the baby.

It is occasionally necessary for a pregnant woman to have her pelvis measured by means of X-rays. There may be certain indications of the need for this in pregnancy and labour but it is for the doctor to decide when this special examination should be arranged. If required, this examination is carried out later in pregnancy when the risks to the baby are much reduced.

Advice in Pregnancy

The mother will be told at the ante-natal clinic how to take care of herself and what special things she should do or not do during pregnancy. Here we give you general advice only. If there is any doubt about anything, your own doctor knows your case best and should be consulted about it. Never feel that a problem is too trivial or sounds silly. If it worries you, discuss it with your doctor or midwife.

Exercise. Vigorous exercise should be stopped, particularly during the early months when there is a tendency to miscarry. The best and safest exercise is walking. Cycling, swimming or gardening can be continued, provided this is not vigorous and you are used to it. If your employment involves much standing you should leave this during the last few months of pregnancy. Many employers will be sympathetic to the situation and it may be possible to change or modify your job to remove some of the physical burden.

Clothes. It is important to avoid wearing rolled stockings, belts, or anything which constricts the body or limbs. Clothes should be such that they hang loosely and avoid pressure on the abdomen. Maternity clothes are now smarter and better designed than before. Take the advice of a local clothing store which specializes in this field or use one of the big mail-order firms which deal exclusively in this type of business. Their catalogues are a mine of information about what you can get for yourself and the baby. The old sack-like uniform of pregnancy has been replaced by smart suits, dresses and sensible underwear.

Intercourse. Many couples avoid sexual intercourse during early pregnancy – up to the tenth week – but it does not seem to carry any risk even as late as the last weeks, provided there has been no bleeding in pregnancy. In later pregnancy the size and shape of the woman's abdomen may be a barrier but this can be overcome by a change of position by the couple.

Rest. Ideally an hour's rest should be taken in bed every afternoon in the second half of pregnancy (see p. 40). Before this, try to rest after the midday meal, with your shoes off and your feet raised on a chair. If you can lie down you will find that you probably drop off to sleep in a little time. Whenever you are sitting down try to get your feet up.

Appearance. Some women find that the condition of their hair deteriorates in pregnancy and that they get spots on the face. The hormone alterations at this time are conducive to increased oiliness of the skin and so more attention should be given to your normal toilet procedures. Use cleansing creams and wash your hair as you would have done before pregnancy, and certainly not less frequently.

Bathing. If it is not possible to have a bath each day, then a sponge-down should be arranged. Personal cleanliness is essential, particularly of the vulva and vagina. Douching may be dangerous and should not be practised.

Breasts. Care of the breasts during pregnancy is important since this helps successful breast-feeding later. The nipples may not be as prominent as they should be; with proper instruction from your midwife and by wearing special shells inside the brassiere it is possible to help the nipples become more prominent and easier for the baby to grip. It is usual for your medical attendant to examine your breasts early in pregnancy and to decide whether such treatment is required.

There may be a slight secretion from the breasts in early pregnancy. This should be cleansed away each day by washing the nipples with ordinary soap and water, using a soft piece of cotton wool for drying. A well-fitting brassiere is naturally part of the care of the breasts. The straps should be wide (about one inch) and the breasts should be supported underneath but not compressed. A brassiere that hooks up in the centre may be an advantage but this depends on the size of the breasts. Take the advice of your doctor or midwife about this.

Diet. It used to be thought that a pregnant woman should eat for two. One of these two is a child who even at birth is only a twentieth of the mother's weight; it must be realized that the second person for whom she is advised to eat requires very little even if he is growing rapidly. If she does eat for two, the mother will put on weight which will be very difficult to lose later.

Most ante-natal clinics give advice on individual diets, but generally speaking the mother should remember to eat body-building substances (proteins) and avoid the weight-increasing substances (carbohydrates). Extra energy will be required in pregnancy because of the extra weight to be carried but only a little of what is eaten is required for that. The real need at this time is for materials which will build the baby's body and the tissues of your own supporting system. These come from the protein foods (meat, fish and cheese), which should be eaten in good quantities. Eggs also provide protein but eaten in large amounts do tend to constipate some people.

In addition to these foods, essential minerals and vitamins are required for the growth of the unborn child. The most important among these are vitamin A (found in highly-coloured fruit and vegetables), vitamin C (in leafy vegetables, tomatoes and citrus fruits), vitamin D (in oily fish and butter), folic acid (in fresh green vegetables and liver), calcium for normal bone-building (best found in milk, cheese and tinned fish), and iron to make blood and provide stores for the future (found in liver, meat and red wine). A woman who has a reasonably well-balanced diet in this country will have plenty of the correct vitamins and minerals in her food and will not usually require extra supplements except for iron and folic acid as mentioned previously. Salt intake is probably best kept to moderation levels, adding it to the cooking as usual but limiting the amount taken at meals.

It always used to be considered good to drink a lot of milk in pregnancy. A pint of milk a day is quite enough and two pints is not twice as good. Too much milk causes the mother to put on weight and, while it is a good fluid food in moderation, much of its goodness can be obtained from other less fattening food sources.

Smoking. Smoking cigarettes undoubtedly affects the unborn child. A heavy smoker (one who smokes more than twenty cigarettes a day) is liable to produce a baby who will be smaller in birth weight for any given period of pregnancy than a woman who does not smoke. Smoking affects health adversely and so should be kept to a minimum anyway, but in pregnancy it should be reduced because it is not just the mother's health that is being affected but that of the unborn child. If a woman gives up smoking in the first few months of pregnancy the baby will be nearer the normal expected weight than if she had continued heavy smoking throughout pregnancy.

Alcohol. There is no harm, however, in drinking in moderation during pregnancy though some women find they develop an aversion to alcohol at this time.

Teeth. As mentioned before, any dental decay can spread more rapidly in pregnancy. Visit your dentist during the first few months to correct anything already in need of attention and go for another check in the last three months (see p. 49).

Heartburn and indigestion. The burning feeling in the lower chest and throat is due to acid from the stomach being pushed up into the rather more delicate oesophagus or gullet where it burns. This usually happens in late pregnancy when the woman is lying down or bending forwards. It can be cured by correct posture, for example sleeping propped up on four or five pillows arranged to support the back, the neck and the head. In an acute situation, alkali mixtures may be used to help reduce pain and, if none of these are easily available, half a glass of milk will make the situation more comfortable.

Bowels. Bowel action can be maintained regularly by eating the proper food, which should consist of liberal amounts of fruits, roughage, vegetables and fresh salads. See that you drink plenty of fluids and, if you are used to taking a laxative, continue to do so, but take medical advice before starting to use a new or stronger one in pregnancy.

Piles. The veins which surround the lower part of the back passage can become engorged and may protrude through the anus. These are piles and are particularly common in pregnancy when the pelvis is filled by the growing baby. They can be reduced in severity by preventing constipation and by ensuring that there is a regular motion each day. Should the discomfort become really unpleasant a soothing ointment or foam can be prescribed by your doctor. Usually piles get much smaller when the pregnancy is over.

Varicose veins. The smaller veins in the legs take extra pressure when there is a mass of uterus and baby distending the abdomen and pressing on the larger veins as they pass through the pelvis. In consequence, varicose veins do appear more commonly in pregnancy at the back of the calves and the inside of the thighs. These may take the form of soft knots sticking through the skin or may simply cause a blue discoloration. When pregnancy is over a lot of the varicosity goes away but often some is left. The discomfort of varicose veins during pregnancy can be controlled by elasticated stockings, or better still, by tights, but this does not cure the problem. The veins are either self-cured when pregnancy is over or may require treatment by injection or surgery later.

Cramps. Some women may feel cramps in the abdomen or calves of the legs in pregnancy. In the abdomen they are common in early and mid pregnancy as the uterus rises up from the pelvis stretching its supporting ligaments. Later on the uterus may press on to the nerves going from the back of the pelvis to the leg and cause a sciatica pain moving from the buttocks down the back of the leg to the foot. The best treatment is to lie down on the side so that the baby may be lifted off the pressure point.

Many pregnant women get cramp in the calves, particularly in bed at night time when the legs warm up. These pains can usually be relieved by rubbing and massaging the affected muscles.

Posture. The pelvis is the basin of bone made by the two hips and the bottom of the spine. It can be tilted into various positions. When you lie on the floor and arch your back the rim or 'brim' of the basin moves forward. When you stand the weight of your baby tends to tilt your pelvis forward in the same way and the arch in your back increases because you have to lean your body backwards to keep a balance. This is quite natural and it will only cause backache if the pelvis is allowed to tilt forward too far. It may happen if you are overtired, when the fine balance of the muscles which hold the pelvis may be upset. It is therefore wise to avoid standing for long periods and to sit down with the feet up whenever possible, particularly when doing household tasks like preparing vegetables. A healthy active woman who moves freely may not have posture problems. Modern advice on weight control in pregnancy has done much to lessen the likelihood of backache but if it should arise seek the advice of your clinic, where you will be shown how to stand and move so as to redistribute your weight and put less unnatural strain on your muscles and ligaments. In many clinics now classes are given during pregnancy by trained physiotherapists who can teach you the way to stand and use your muscles properly.

Relaxation. Pregnancy and labour can be uncomfortable but as well as getting pain relief from medicaments and drugs some women gain great benefit from relaxation exercises, which reduce discomfort and conserve energy. The easiest way to learn relaxation is to practise it repeatedly in the privacy of your home. Many helpful classes are run and the instructors at these can give guidance but the basic learning still comes from repeated practice. Here we give only a brief outline, for this is best learned from practical instruction.

Before settling down to your practice, you should remove your shoes and loosen your clothes. It is probably best to lie on the floor and make yourself comfortable. Two positions are the most popular, on the back with a pillow under the head and knees, or on the side with the legs drawn up, the top one bent over a pillow and a little more flexed than the other. This is a position in which all the joints of the body are flexed. Some women find relaxation practice in late pregnancy is more easily achieved in the upright position for they can concentrate better and breathing is not so encumbered. It is best to try both and use the position found to be more comfortable.

The idea of these exercises is to show the contrast between relaxation and tension of the muscles. Start by working on one arm only. Rest the arm on the floor, clench your fist, then loosen it. Repeat this a few times. Each time you clench your fist you will notice the feeling in your forearm produced by muscle tension. You must learn to recognize this sensation. When you loosen your fist you relax the muscles of your forearm and you should also notice this feeling carefully. Thus you will learn to contrast the sensation of tension and relaxation. It is fairly easy in the limbs, but as you gain practice and work systematically through your body, you will be able to notice the same kind of feeling in other parts – for instance, in the neck, the back and the face.

Beginning with one arm, first practise with the fist, then with the elbow, making it straight and stiff; then shrug the shoulders hard, in each case first tensing and then relaxing, carefully noticing the difference between the two sensations. Repeat all this on the other arm. Next work on the legs in the same way. Turn up the feet as far as they will go and then let them drop; press the knees firmly on the floor and then slacken them; finally, squeeze the buttocks together and then relax them.

After that you must find the tensions in your trunk: this is more difficult. If you raise the middle of your back off the floor and then let it sink again you will feel some tension in the neck. Neck muscles are often tense. Press your head back and then relax; raise your head and then let it go. The face is the most difficult to relax. Shut your eyes very tightly and then let go. All expression depends on some muscle tension. You must not mind letting your face go vacant. Place the tip of your tongue behind the upper front teeth and let the jaw drop. Your jaw muscles must relax as well as the rest; when this is done your chin will drop.

If you want to learn other exercises your best plan is to spend at least half an hour each day cultivating this ability to relax your muscles. Once you have learnt about tensions you will begin relaxing immediately without going through the preliminary exercises. As you become good at it you will quickly feel completely at ease. After your relaxation practice, do not jump up too quickly or you may get giddy. Stretch yourself out slowly, until you feel the blood filling up your limbs again. As well as your specific half hour's practice, watch yourself at various times during the day. When the opportunity allows, sit back and let the muscles loosen within the limitations allowed.

Breathing exercises. Breathing patterns will change as pregnancy advances and the baby gets bigger, pushing up on the underside of the diaphragm (see Figure 12). Many women find that certain types of breathing exercises give much relief, particularly during labour. You should practise deep breathing, lying on your back with your knees bent and your feet placed apart. Put your hands on your abdomen and breathe in deeply and slowly so that you can feel the abdomen rise. Then breathe out slowly, feeling your abdomen sink. Do it about a dozen times in a steady rhythmical way. This is the kind of breathing which will be of great help to you in the first stage of labour when you are feeling the contractions of the uterus.

As labour progresses and the second stage approaches, then you will find that abdominal breathing no longer helps you and that you are automatically breathing in the upper part of your chest. You can prepare for this, in the weeks before labour, in the following way. Continue to keep your attention on the rhythm of breathing. Many women find it helpful to 'breathe in threes'. Take three small, almost imperceptible breaths in and out through the mouth; repeat this grouping so long as the pain lasts and concentrate on relaxing when it is over. It is important to keep the eyes open and concentrate on some object in the room, such as a clock on the wall. This 'breathing in threes' technique can be practised in the weeks before labour, when painless but easily felt contractions of the uterus are noticed. Do not attempt noisy overbreathing for this does not help. Quiet, deep rhythmical efforts are useful, great gasps are not.

When you move well into the second stage of labour you will, of course, need another type of breathing for pushing down. You will have to take a deep breath, hold it, and press down as hard as you can as though you were pushing your anus through the bed. Your body will do this of its own accord and you will not need much practice.

Finally, there is a shallow sort of panting breathing which many doctors and midwives will like you to use when the baby's head is nearly delivered (see p. 71). But do not trouble about what you must do at the time of the birth: your midwife or doctor will tell you exactly. Neither relaxation nor control of breathing will guarantee you a painless labour, but they are effective ways by which you can help yourself reduce pain and conserve energy.

There are organizations which give practical instruction in these methods. If your doctor agrees, contact the local branch of one of them. But even such simple methods as have been briefly described above produce results so convincing to those who have seriously tried them that they can be recommended with confidence.

Social Security benefits. These are available to most pregnant women and are paid by the government. Details are in a leaflet available at your ante-natal clinic and if you have any doubts, you should speak to the medical social worker there.

A maternity grant (£25) can be obtained if you or your husband have paid twenty-six flat rate contributions to the National Insurance. A form to apply for this grant can be obtained by applying to your local Social Security office, or your ante-natal clinic. Should you have twins, the maternity grant is doubled.

A maternity allowance of £8.60 a week is paid for

eighteen weeks before the child is due and eleven weeks after its birth. It is paid to working mothers who have themselves paid the twenty-six National Insurance contributions within the year immediately preceding the fourteenth week before the birth of the child. It will be affected if you are working or receiving some other benefit from the government. This too can be claimed from the local Social Security office by sending in a certificate of expected confinement from your doctor or midwife. Details of these financial grants will alter with variations in the coming months and years. Check with your medical social worker what the current situation is and read the leaflets provided.

Up to seven pints of free milk a week can be obtained by mothers who have two other children under school age or by those in families receiving supplementary benefits or family income supplements. This benefit can be continued after the baby is born.

During pregnancy and for a year after delivery, dental treatment is free to women and during pregnancy itself any N.H.S. prescription charges are waived.

Chapter 6

DELIVERY OF THE BABY

WHEN a woman reaches the expected date of her delivery she may get impatient because there are no signs of labour. It must be remembered that the mathematical chances are that the baby will probably not come exactly on this day but a little before or after. It does not matter if nothing happens on this date for its calculation has been very approximate. Its real purpose has been to give guidance and to mark out to within a week or so the time when the child may be born. Ninety per cent of babies will come within ten days on either side of this given date but the other ten per cent may come earlier or later.

The Mother's View of Labour

Labour can start in several different ways but there are certain general patterns.

The early signs of labour may be:
  (1) Painful, intermittent regular contractions of the uterus.
  (2) A 'show' or loss of a slight bloodstained discharge.
  (3) The rupture of the membranes – the breaking of the waters.

When any of the above signs occur, it means that labour has started and that you should get in touch with your hospital or, if delivery is to be at home, with your midwife.

There is a very important difference between women having their first baby and those who have had one before. The first group may have uncomfortable uterine contractions for several days or even weeks before labour starts. If they are in any doubt, they should contact their hospital but it is probably safe to wait until the contractions are felt every fifteen minutes or so. Such women are probably not going to produce the baby in a few minutes and so this should be about the correct time to go into hospital.

It is notoriously more difficult to assess women who have had a baby before. Often a previous boring and unnecessary stay in hospital for a few days has made them chary of moving too soon in the current pregnancy. They want to stay with their family until they are sure that they really are in labour. Our best advice to them is that, knowing that they could deliver more speedily than when the first baby was coming, they should go to hospital as soon as the contractions become regular (every twenty minutes or so). Only in this way can they be sure of getting to the hospital in time to benefit from its specialized attention. Of course if there is a show of blood or the membranes rupture this will be an indication to any mother that she should go to hospital immediately.

1. UTERINE CONTRACTIONS

Often these contractions are mistaken for colic. A mother will say: 'I thought it was some gooseberries that I ate', mistakenly thinking that it is the intestine and not the uterus that is contracting. You may well have already noticed some contractions during pregnancy and have felt the uterus harden. With the onset of labour an ache develops in the small of the back as you have one of these contractions. The ache will at first be localized to the lower part of the back and, as labour progresses, it will radiate round to the front. When you feel a contraction coming down to the front, put a hand on your abdomen and you will feel the uterus hardening. This is muscle working like any other muscle.

DELIVERY OF THE BABY

If you clench your fist and bend your elbow firmly, your biceps will harden and stand up. It is exactly the same with the uterus. When a muscle works it does so by shortening itself and if it goes on doing this for some time it begins to ache. It is in this way that the contractions of labour differ from the contractions of pregnancy. Whilst the former are painless, with the latter you will feel an ache.

The contractions of the uterus at first come once or twice an hour, then every twenty minutes. Later, the intervals become shorter until eventually they occur every two minutes. 'False labour' is a condition when the contractions start, reach a certain frequency and then become less and pass off completely. This false alarm may start a week or so before real labour begins. The presence of a 'show' sometimes helps to differentiate false from true labour.

2. THE SHOW

The small amount of bloodstained mucus which may be passed at the onset of labour is due to the opening or dilation of the cervix and the stripping off of a little of the membrane stuck to its inner side. If it appears the mother should contact the hospital and be prepared to go in, for this is a sign of the beginning of the first stage of labour.

3. RUPTURE OF THE MEMBRANES

Occasionally labour may start with an escape of some of the fluid which has been surrounding the baby in the uterus. This is more common in women who have had a baby before and is less likely with the first pregnancy. It happens unexpectedly and a rubber or plastic sheet under the bottom sheet can save a soaked mattress. The amount of fluid lost is variable and it does not mean that if the membranes rupture early you will have a 'dry' and prolonged labour. In many labours, membrane rupture does not occur until late in the first stage and in others the doctor or midwife may rupture them.

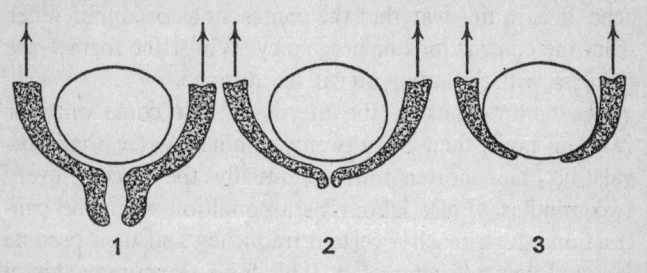

Figure 14 The cervix in labour, showing how the cervix is pulled up from above, dilating the entrance to the uterus.

The first stage of labour. This is the stage of preparation of the birth canal and is measured from the start of labour to the full dilation of the cervix. You will recall how the uterus has been described as a muscular bag with an opening at its lower end. When labour begins (see Figure 14), the sides of this bag start to shorten and pull themselves up. This is followed by a widening and opening of the cervix while at the same time the baby is gradually being pushed downwards. When the cervix is fully open it reaches its maximum width (four inches in diameter) to allow the baby's head to come through. The first stage of labour is now completed. The last part of this stage is the most uncomfortable of the whole of labour. When you have finished this, the worst is over.

Early in labour the mother may wish to carry on gently with some ordinary activity, for example reading. What you do depends partly on your midwife or doctor. But there comes a time when the contractions get stronger and you will prefer to lie down. This is the time when you will find

DELIVERY OF THE BABY

benefit if you have practised relaxation. Let yourself go as loose as possible between the contractions and when they come take deep breaths as has been described (see p. 58). This is a great help but almost as important is your feeling about the whole affair. Fear can make labour more painful. From ancient times the cycle has been recognized of the three sensations felt during the first stage of labour – fear, pain and tension. Any one of these may give rise to the other two. Tension can be reduced by relaxing, fear by knowledge of the events to come and confidence in your doctors and midwives. Decrease of both reduces pain and what remains can be dealt with by properly selected treatments from your doctor.

Fear of the unknown is lessened by the confidence that comes from knowing something about what will happen in labour. If the mother has been receiving some ante-natal instruction she will find that fear will not dominate her behaviour at this time. Mothers react in various ways when it comes to labour, but all agree that being forewarned gives them tremendous confidence. Sometimes an irrational fear seizes us and this is difficult to argue ourselves out of. If the mind affects the body it also follows that the body can affect the mind. These sort of fears can often be best fought off by concentrating on steady breathing and relaxing the muscles. Some mothers get help in concentrating their minds away from the present situation by tapping out a popular tune with their fingers against their own abdomen and watching their fingers while this is going on. Others take the philosophical point of view of dealing with each contraction as it comes; when it is over that is one more out of the way and one less to come. Whatever aids you use, now is the time when you want to try to maintain a calm and anxiety-free attitude towards labour.

There are two more things which will help the mother at

this time and, although they appear to be opposites, they work together. The first is the need for self-discipline, the second the need to give herself up to what is happening – to let herself go. Self-discipline means realizing that she herself is in some way responsible for the kind of labour she will have. Labour means hard work – your baby will not be delivered without some effort on your part. This does not mean that you will not have every help science can give you. In recent years the relief of pain in labour has become a subject to which much research is devoted. Many drugs and techniques are now available and the one best suited to your own needs, given by your doctor in your own hospital, will be used to help you. Further, medical research is concentrating on helping the unborn child. Doctors and midwives can now tell a lot more about the baby inside the uterus and many tests and observations will be used to keep your baby well during the hours of labour. However, in the long run it is the mother who has to go through the work of labour and scientific advances cannot do much more than assist her and her unborn child. If you remember this, then you will not expect science to produce your baby for you and you will not be disappointed. If you are disappointed you might get frightened, and if frightened give yourself needless trouble and pain.

The other helpful attitude in labour is to give yourself up to a process that is inevitable. If anything goes amiss, that would be the concern of the doctor or midwife. There is nothing you can do except give them your confidence. Be prepared to accept the help given and do not be too adamant in refusing pain relief if your medical helpers think it would be useful. Otherwise let yourself work with nature. Nature will have her way in the end so it is much easier to co-operate.

Transition of first to second stage. As you get near the end of the first stage you may notice other things happening within yourself. You may begin to feel shivery or hot; if the membranes are still intact they will now break – perhaps rather suddenly; you may feel as though you want to open your bowels and you may pass a little blood from the vagina. This is the boring time when the sensation of something filling the pelvis leads to an almost irresistible desire to push the baby out. Since the cervix – neck of the womb – may not yet be fully dilated, this would be unhelpful and it takes a lot of self-restraint to prevent bearing down. Again, it is best to be guided by your advisers, who will give you the pain relief best suited to you and your unborn child's safety.

The second stage. This is the stage of expulsion – measured from the full dilation of the cervix to delivery of the baby. You will know that you are approaching the second stage when you feel a pressure on the back passage as though you want to open your bowels. Presently, with each contraction, you will get a strong urge to bear down, making use of your abdominal muscles to help press your baby out. You should get the agreement of your doctor or midwife before you do this for you must not bear down too early.

You will find it a great relief when you begin to push. Nearly all women describe the comfort received in taking an active part in the delivery of their baby, having put behind them the more passive hours of the first stage. It is important to do this pushing properly, and if you have been trained you will know how to get the maximum effect from pushing at the time of the contraction of the uterus. When you feel a contraction coming, take a few quick breaths in and out and then hold your breath and push steadily, keeping up the pressure for ten to fifteen seconds (see p. 59). Then repeat the procedure, pausing only long enough to take another lungful of air, until the contraction is over. Then let yourself go quite limp and take a rest – you will need it, for

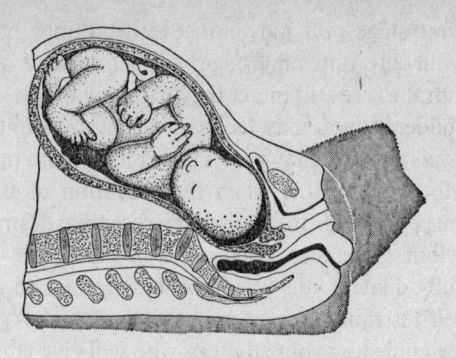

Figure 15 The stages in labour.

(a) *The uterus in late pregnancy*. This baby is lying in the uterus facing the right side of the mother with his arms and legs flexed against his body. He has descended a little into the mother's pelvis. The cervix is still long and unripe; the membranes are still intact and the pelvic floor is still thick.

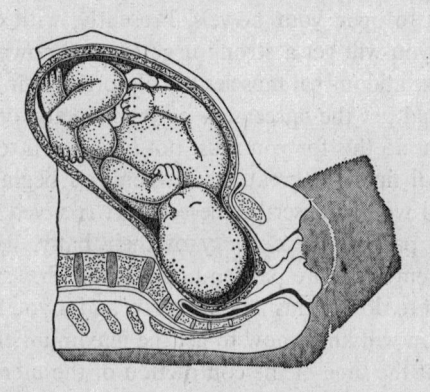

(b) *Just before labour or in early labour*. The cervix has now been pulled up and no longer has a canal but it has not yet started to dilate very much. This may happen in the latter days of pregnancy or in early labour itself. The membranes are still intact, and the bag of forewaters is being formed in front of the baby's head. The head is being flexed more against the chest so as to provide as small a diameter as possible to pass through the pelvis.

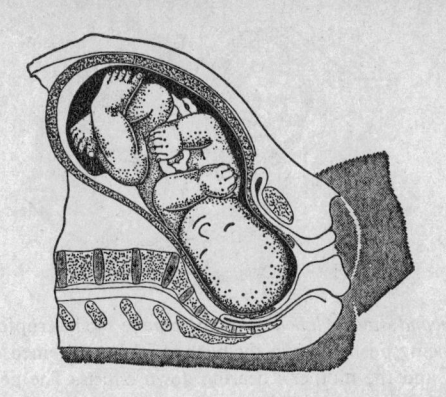

(c) *The first stage of labour*. The cervix has now been completely effaced and is dilating; the bag of forewaters is bulging through the cervix. The uterus is contracting, pushing the baby's head further down into the mother's pelvis.

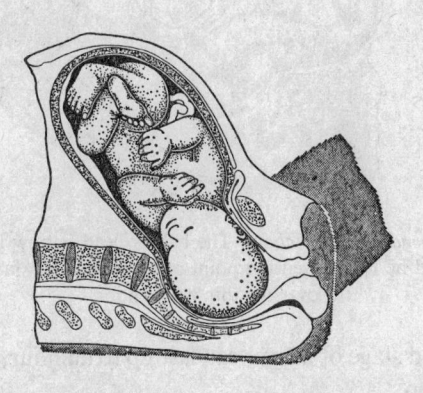

(d) *The end of the first stage of labour*. The cervix is now fully dilated and the baby's head is filling the pelvis. The bag of forewaters has usually ruptured by this time but in this particular diagram is still present. The vagina and the uterus are now one tube.

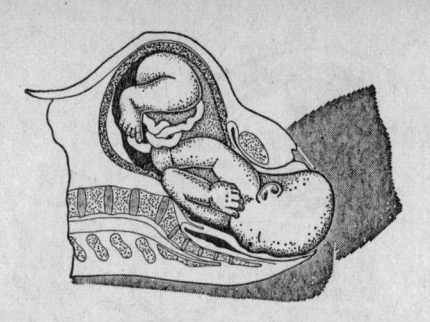

(e) *The second stage of labour.* The membrane sac has ruptured and the baby is being pushed down the birth canal by combined uterine contractions and the mother's bearing down efforts. The pelvic floor is very thin and the baby's head can be seen protruding between the lips of the vulva.

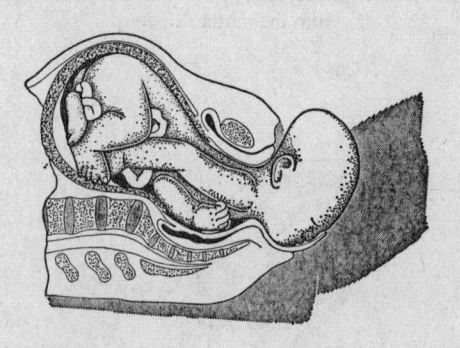

(f) *The second stage of labour.* The baby's head is now beginning to emerge and he has passed the point of no return. His face is passing over the thin pelvic floor.

the second stage of labour can last up to an hour, often less, rarely more.

When the baby is nearly ready to be born you feel your muscles stretching – this is another time when you may feel uncomfortable. Many mothers say that it is not nearly so

DELIVERY OF THE BABY

much a feeling of pain as of anxiety – wondering what is going to happen next. It is nothing like the pain felt earlier at the end of the first stage. This is another time when it will help if you have practised letting your muscles go by relaxation. Just let your baby come. Push down a little when you are asked. Stop pushing and pant when you are later asked to do that.

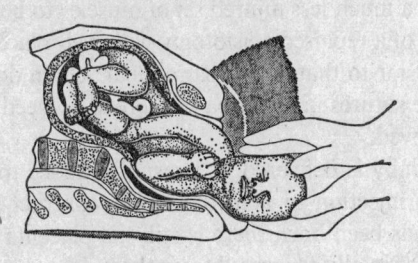

(g) *The delivery of the head.* The head, the largest and hardest part of the baby, has now been born. He has rotated and the hands of the obstetrician are guiding the head. The shoulders have entered the pelvis and the body is rotating round to allow their passage. At this stage the placenta will start to separate but will not be delivered until after the baby has been born.

It is sometimes possible for the mother to see her baby born if her head and shoulders are raised up on pillows. She will be pushing her baby out still further under the direction of her doctor or midwife. It is very important to pay attention to the midwife's instructions at this stage for when the baby's head is about to be born it is advisable for the mother to stop further pushing. This prevents the baby from being born at a rush for if he were he could damage the vulva and the tissues at the lower end of the vagina. Many doctors and midwives, when looking after mothers at this stage, ask them to stop pushing just as the baby's head reaches the floor of the vagina. They ask the mother to breathe rapidly and it is important that she should stop pushing when instructed.

Another way of reducing the damage that stretch can do to the muscles and tissues of the pelvic floor is to make a clean surgical division under local anaesthetic. This is an episiotomy; all midwives and doctors are trained to perform this small operation to prevent the worst tears which can occur at the lower end of the vagina. It is usually hardly felt, and leaves a much less injured set of muscles to be repaired. The result of a repaired episiotomy with well-placed stitches is far superior to that of a repaired tear. Often doctors use absorbable sutures in this area so there is no need for them to be removed.

As the baby is delivered, it is usual practice to give the mother an injection to help the uterus contract, for after the baby has been born there is still the placenta to come. The baby is usually separated from the mother by clamping and tying the umbilical cord. This is not painful to the baby, for there are no nerves in this cord.

The third stage. This is the time taken for the expulsion of the placenta. Although the baby is born, there is still this last event to complete, but it is only a small piece of work on the mother's part. You will recall that the placenta is attached to the wall of the uterus. It will now have separated and there may be a small gush of blood from the vagina. You will at this time feel the contractions return in a very mild way and you may be asked to push out the placenta, or the doctor or midwife may deliver it for you by steadying the uterus through the abdominal wall and gently tensing the umbilical cord so that the placenta is drawn down from the uterus.

These are the processes of labour. The duration of each stage varies according to whether it is a first or subsequent delivery. The first labour will naturally last longer than subsequent ones – most women may expect it to last between eight and twenty hours.

The Management of Labour

The description just given is an attempt to explain the mother's reactions and sensations. At the same time, doctors and midwives have various tasks to do to make labour safer and more comfortable. For instance, some hospitals still give an enema early in labour. Soapy water washes out the rectum so as to empty the lower bowel and help the progress of labour by increasing the force of the contractions. The genital hair may either be shaved or clipped closely. This is part of the normal hygiene of labour and for the same reason it is a good idea for the mother to have a bath or spongedown. She will be encouraged to move around or to lie down whenever she feels like it.

Food. With the increased activity of muscles during labour there is more demand upon the mother's energy, but it is a mistake for her to eat and drink too much during this time. Often mothers lose their appetite and there may even be a tendency to vomit for the usual propulsion mechanisms of the stomach and intestines are greatly diminished during labour. Hence any food taken might not be passed on to where it is going to be digested but instead may remain in the stomach as an undigested mass. It is far better to drink fluids and follow a light diet as guided by the hospital or midwife. Mothers should remember that labour is not going to go on for very long and that any reduction in eating is only for a short time.

Sleep. The amount of sleep to be had at this time depends on when labour starts. It is better to feel refreshed and rested as much as possible, for lying awake at night in early labour is not desirable. The mother is therefore often given sedatives in the form of tablets or injections to help her have a more natural sleep. After a few hours' rest she will feel much stronger for the work that lies ahead.

Relief of pain (analgesia). Uterine contractions can be painful, particularly during the first stage of labour. It is common practice in this country to give pain-relieving drugs during this stage. By far the commonest of these is pethidine, a powerful pain-stopping drug which also relieves tension and prevents spasm of the uterine muscle. It is usually given by injection into the buttocks and may take fifteen to twenty minutes to start working so do not expect immediate relief. One pethidine injection will last two to four hours and make life much more bearable without making the patient unconscious. The giving of pain-relieving drugs must be left to the discretion of the midwife or doctor in charge of the individual case. Often the attendant will want to make sure that labour has started properly before giving any such analgesics, for if given too early they could postpone the uterine contractions and so prolong labour.

Mention has already been made of the most painful part of labour as being the transition between the first and second stages, just before the mother feels an irresistible desire to start bearing down. It is now that she may require some additional aid in the form of inhalation analgesia. At present two agents are commonly used, nitrous oxide and trilene. They each come in simple-to-use equipment controlled by the mother, who has usually been shown how to handle it during the ante-natal period. She should have been told how to take deep breaths of either the gas mixed with oxygen or of the trilene and then use her diaphragm and abdominal muscles to help push her baby down when the doctor or midwife advises. It is interesting to note that, during the second stage, when the mother wishes to bear down, the lower part of the vagina and perineum is partly anaesthe-

DELIVERY OF THE BABY

tized. It seems that the act of pushing is in itself a pain-relieving manoeuvre provided the mother knows how to do it. It is, of course, hard work, but that does not mean to say that it is painful.

The next phase when pain may be felt is when the head presses on the lower vagina. Anxiety is often a major factor when the mother fears that she is going to damage or split the tissues of the vulva at the entrance of the vagina. She need not feel this anxiety since the birth of the head is properly controlled by the attendant. Local anaesthetic is often injected into the tissues to relieve unpleasant sensations. Again, it is at this stage that gas and oxygen or trilene may be given to provide some pain relief without reducing consciousness, for many mothers prefer to be fully awake at the time of the actual delivery of the baby.

In the present day, more powerful methods of pain relief in labour are being used as epidural analgesia is becoming more popular. Here a local anaesthetic agent is injected around the nerves as they pass from the spinal cord towards the pelvis. It must be stressed that it is not a spinal anaesthetic and that the injection is not put into the spinal sac but into the tissues around the spine where the nerves are passing. Such an analgesic relieves pain very effectively throughout labour and delivery. It can be given by an injection in the back, which may be repeated, or a small polythene tube can be led into the area through which repeated injections can be given, thus saving the mother a lot of inconvenience. There are very few side effects of epidural anaesthesia, which is much safer than spinal anaesthetics where problems occasionally arise. The major difficulty with such epidural anaesthesia is that it must be applied by a skilled person, preferably an anaesthetist. Such doctors are only available in the larger maternity units at the moment – small hospitals, general practitioner units and doctors or midwives performing deliveries in the home cannot usually make use of this service. Indeed, such is the shortage of doctors in hospitals at the moment that even many of the larger maternity units cannot always promise this facility. When the staff are available such a means of pain relief gives the mother a very good labour and the baby a very good chance of starting life in an unstressed state.

Other methods of relieving pain have been put to the test by many mothers with excellent results. However much medical science helps, most agree that the better trained a mother is for her delivery the more she can help herself during labour, with or without the aid of analgesia. It must be understood that it is not a confession of failure if a mother has analgesia, no matter what degree of training or preparation for childbirth she may have experienced. There are some women who, having attended some classes at antenatal clinics, feel that by asking for an analgesic drug they are letting down the side. This is not so. The analgesic drugs assist anything she may have learned. Having a baby is a matter of team work, in which the most important member of the team is the mother. If she has full confidence in her attendants, this will help her let herself go and relieve any mental tension she may have had before the delivery. If she is aware of the changes taking place during the process of birth she will recognize these and look upon them as milestones along the road to her ultimate delivery. Labour can be made a most satisfying and exhilarating experience with the aid of modern scientific methods. No woman should ever deny herself, or be denied, any of the available methods of pain relief when she requires them.

Vaginal examination. You will probably have several internal examinations in labour. Such investigations are necessary to show the doctor or midwife how labour is progressing, how the cervix is opening to allow the passage of the baby,

DELIVERY OF THE BABY

how far the baby's head has come down in the pelvic cavity and whether the bag of membranes is intact or not. You will also have a lot of abdominal examinations at intervals, to check the position and descent of the baby, and his heart will be listened to and recorded on a chart. This is all part of the routine management of labour.

Care of the bladder. Often there is a tendency for the bladder to fill and for the mother to have difficulty in passing water during labour. This has to be carefully watched and it may be necessary to have a catheter passed. This is not painful and by relieving the retention of urine, the progress of labour is expedited.

Induced labour. While most women start their labour naturally, about a quarter of them will have it started by their doctors. Labour will be induced for reasons which may be concerned with the mother or the maintenance of her unborn baby's health. In this country induction may be done either by stimulating the uterus with hormone substances or by breaking the waters around the baby, while some hospitals use a combination of these methods. The hormones may be given to the woman to suck so that they are absorbed into the blood vessels of the cheek and so circulate around the blood. The alternative method is to introduce the hormones directly into the blood stream by means of an intravenous drip inserted into a small vein in the arm. In either case the uterus is soon stimulated into action. The waters around the baby can be gently punctured through the cervix or neck of the womb by the doctor. This is rather like a vaginal examination and is just as painless. Since labour is obviously close, very often full sterile precautions are taken during the puncture of the membranes. Either method of induction is usually followed by labour fairly quickly.

In this country most doctors do not recommend induction of labour for convenience, and will do so only when there are medical reasons. The commonest of these are the conditions of pre-eclampsia (discussed in Chapter 9), or when the baby stays inside the uterus for a prolonged time. This will be discussed with you by your doctor.

Operative Deliveries

Nine out of ten women who read this book will have a normal delivery but a small number require assistance in order to have a healthy baby. Occasionally babies show signs of a reduction in their oxygen supply during labour and the doctor may consider it wise to accelerate delivery. This usually results in a forceps delivery, when a pair of carefully constructed guides are placed on either side of the baby's head in order to help delivery from the vagina. This sounds a formidable procedure but nowadays it always takes place with some form of anaesthetic (either a general one or by injection to numb the nerves of the pelvis) and most women experience no more pain with a forceps delivery than they do with a normal one. The forceps blades themselves are very skilfully designed and have been tested by centuries of use. They are moulded to slip into position easily and have a limited closing action, thus protecting the baby's head and not squeezing it. Forceps are used only if they are necessary to help produce a healthy baby.

An even smaller number of women may have a Caesarean section. This is an operative delivery whereby the baby is delivered by incision low down on the stomach wall and through the uterus. This is only performed if it is essential for the health of the mother or baby and takes place under a general anaesthetic with the mother completely asleep. It causes a certain amount of discomfort for the subsequent few days but is not a terribly painful procedure and, again, the end result of a healthy mother and baby justifies the operation.

Chapter 7

POST-NATAL CARE

THE lying-in period comes immediately after the delivery and has no well-defined length. It is conventionally taken as the time a woman spends in hospital after childbirth while she is starting the recovery process. Her organs are now beginning to return to their pre-pregnancy state and she is learning to deal with the baby. When delivery has been in hospital, a mother stays in the lying-in ward for about seven days, but in some centres this is extended to ten days. In a few units, as has been mentioned previously, a planned early discharge can be arranged, the mother having her delivery in hospital and being sent home to the care of her family doctor and midwife within forty-eight hours. This is a facility which has to be arranged well in advance during the pregnancy so that the community medical and nursing services know the patient is coming under their care. Should the delivery be at home the mother will usually stay in bed for some days after childbirth: in this case the demarcation line between lying in and convalescence is much less rigid for the mother will obviously join in the activities of the household in a more gradual way.

A different term used for the time after delivery is the puerperium, from the Latin *puer* (child) and *parere* (to bear). This is the time allowed for the recovery process of the mother's organs. The muscles of the abdominal wall, the pelvic floor and the uterus take much more than the seven to ten days of the lying-in period to resume their pre-pregnant condition. Conventionally in this country the puerperium is considered to be about six weeks. By the end of this time not all the body tissues have returned to their pre-pregnant state, but the majority of women have regained their normal activities and the body has adapted itself after the birth of the child. Thus it is usual to differentiate between the lying-in period and the longer puerperium.

The uterus. Immediately after the baby is born the uterus weighs about two pounds and has a length of twelve inches and a breadth of eight inches. Before pregnancy, the uterus weighed two ounces and was two and a half inches long. Each muscle fibre is now ten times longer and five times thicker than in the non-pregnancy state. The process of returning to the non-pregnant resting state takes time and is known as involution. It consists of a reduction in the size and number of muscle fibres as well as diminution of the blood supply. The uterus will never return to the size it was before pregnancy, but will always be a little bulkier because of the fibrous tissue which is laid down in the uterine wall.

Vaginal discharge (*lochia*). The discharge from the uterus after delivery consists mainly of blood. At first it is red, changing over some days successively to pink, brown, yellow or white. These colour changes represent the expulsion of old blood (some bleeding takes place in the cavity of the uterus at the time of delivery and the blood is slowly expelled from the body in the next few weeks). At first the loss will obviously be near to normal blood colour but as it ages, like a bruise, it undergoes colour changes and fades. The amount and duration varies according to the individual. There may be some red or pink colouration for a few weeks: this is nothing to worry about. If at any time the lochia becomes greater or smells offensive, this should be reported to the doctor. Similarly, he should also be told if there is bright red bleeding once the colour has started to fade.

The breasts. The breasts are developing throughout pregnancy in preparation for lactation. The milk starts to be produced on the first or the second day after delivery, when the mother will feel distension, or tightness in the breasts. It is important to relieve excessive congestion, and if at any time she notices pain she should report this to the midwife. The first two weeks are important for the establishment of breast-feeding. It is during this time that your baby is learning to feed from the breast and your midwife will give you all the possible help and advice at this critical time. Some general comments on infant feeding are made in the next chapter.

Afterpains. These are due to contractions of the uterus and for some women resemble menstrual pains; others find them stronger, like mini labour pains. They are particularly noticed when the baby is put to the breast and are usually felt more frequently after the second or subsequent delivery. Such pains can be relieved by pain-relieving drugs and gradually cease a week or so after delivery.

Emotional worries. The emotional disturbances that some mothers experience during the lying-in period are difficult to explain. They may find themselves crying suddenly for no reason at all. There may be a feeling of anti-climax after all that has happened during the previous months of pregnancy when the excitement was in the expectancy of the coming birth. Once this has happened, a lot of the highlights seem to be dimmed. Looking back on the delivery may not be as exciting and stimulating as looking forward to it. Most mothers soon get over these short attacks of depression, for they are a normal reaction to a strongly emotional event.

Bladder problems. You will notice that you are passing much more urine than normal. This is due to the excessive amount of water that has been retained in your tissues during pregnancy. During the first twenty-four hours after delivery you may pass as much as eight pints. Very occasionally there can be difficulty in emptying the bladder and so retention of urine develops. Any difficulty of this nature must be reported. You should not go many hours (say ten) without passing water and it is much better to have the bladder emptied by a catheter than to allow it to become distended. Normal function will often be established simply by sitting on a warm bedpan or walking to the lavatory.

Hygiene of the lying-in period. During this time the midwife will attend you and will help you with your personal hygiene. She may swab the vulva with an antiseptic solution although many women now prefer to sit in a salt bath soon after delivery. This is most comforting and helps to keep the vulva clean. Such a bath is best prepared with six to eight inches of warm water and a fistful of kitchen salt mixed in (not the more expensive table salt and it is quite unnecessary to spend money on expensive packets of 'sea salt'). You will be provided with sterile sanitary pads which should be changed from time to time. The soiled ones should not be thrown away but kept for the midwife to inspect should she ask you.

Diet. Diet is important during this phase of rehabilitation since there is an association between the quality of food you eat and your return to normal. Nutritional requirements at this time are as great as during pregnancy. You need particularly to increase protein and fluid intake if you are breast-feeding, for the volume of milk made is very dependent on the latter. There is no harm in satisfying your hunger with extra protein and even increasing carbohydrate intake a little, despite the fact that during pregnancy you should resist the temptation to overeat. The quality of food taken in pregnancy should be maintained – the amount may be increased provided that the carbohydrates are carefully watched and not allowed to dominate the diet.

Bowels. There may be difficulty with the bowels during the first week. No harm results from not passing a motion for two or three days; often during the day or so of labour very little solid food is taken and so there is nothing to pass on. The ritual of purgation should be avoided; liquid paraffin or castor oil need not be taken. A mild laxative, such as senna, syrup of figs or milk of magnesia, may help to establish a normal bowel function but this will only be maintained if there is plenty of roughage in the diet and if you take plenty of fluids. Should constipation be more stubborn than this, ask your doctor or midwife for help rather than just taking stronger purges. There may be some way they can assist you.

Post-natal Exercises and Activity

It is a good idea to start exercises shortly after delivery to restore the tone of the abdominal and pelvic floor muscles. Those who deal with rehabilitation have given much thought to these post-natal exercises, which strengthen overstretched muscles simply and effectively. In addition, breathing exercises and leg movements which have a beneficial effect on the circulation should be performed.

The question of early rising is no longer a controversial one. In most hospitals women now sit out of their bed on the day following delivery as part of an 'early ambulation' policy to improve circulation of blood in the legs. This is important for if the circulation were to become sluggish it might lead to blood clotting in the veins. Early ambulation should not be made an excuse for neglecting post-natal exercises. These should be continued for six to eight weeks after delivery but at no time should the mother undertake exercises which fatigue her. Care should be taken not to overwork muscles and joints which are not yet ready to take the strain. Such exercises are best done after discussing the whole matter with a doctor or trained physiotherapist.

The return to housework should be gradual and for some

weeks every effort must be made to avoid lifting heavy weights or moving furniture. If it is necessary to lift anything, less strain will be thrown on the back if the knees are bent and the back kept straight and then the weight lifted by straightening the legs. Bending forward over the sink or over the baby is one of the commonest ways of developing a weakness in the back leading to chronic backache. In the early days of a baby's life, many of the tasks that a mother performs for him involve bending over (e.g. changing nappies); it is advisable for the baby's toilet area to be arranged at a convenient height. This is not at the level of the mother's hips but somewhere near her midriff. Thus, the mother who spends many hours of the day looking after her child will not lay the seeds of strain in her back. Similarly, it should be possible to arrange for the washing-up bowl to be raised to a higher level to avoid further stooping.

Post-natal Exercises

You would be best advised to follow those exercises which the physiotherapist or midwife gives you. Not all activities suit all people and the following advice is given only for general guidance. The exercises are in two groups and the transition from the early to the later ones should be made only after medical advice.

Early

These exercises are intended for practice in bed during the first few days after delivery. Repeat each one slowly and rhythmically about half a dozen times.

POST-NATAL CARE

Breathing

Place your hands lightly on the lower ribs, gently compress the chest and breathe out slowly, emptying the lungs as completely as possible. Then take in quite a deep breath, expanding the lower part of the lungs which should push the ribs out against your hands.

Feet and legs

Bend and stretch your ankles fully in turn, bend and stretch the toes and then move your feet around in large circles. Tighten the muscles above the knees by pressing the backs of your knees down on to the bed, then relax.

Pelvis

Lie on your back with the knees slightly bent and the soles of the feet on the bed. Tighten the seat muscles and at the same time draw in strongly the muscles of the lower abdomen pressing the lower back on to the bed. Relax both groups of muscles allowing your back to hollow slightly. This exercise should be practised regularly; it helps correct the pelvic tilt and is important in the maintenance of correct posture. If there seems to be no response to your efforts to control the muscles, the physiotherapist may suggest different exercises. Do not worry if you achieve little in the first day or two but practise to educate the muscles. Often the bath is the easiest place to do this.

Pelvic floor muscles

1) Lying on your back with the knees bent and feet flat on the bed, relax everything and concentrate on closing the vagina. You should at the same time feel the anus contract. When you achieve this, relax and repeat the exercise.

2) After this lie on your back and contract the muscles of the pelvic floor by drawing upwards the muscles which close the bowels and the vagina. This movement can be reinforced by breathing out slowly as you pull up. Tighten the muscles for a count of five – then relax slowly and completely. If practised carefully and frequently throughout the day, the tightening up during this exercise will help tone up the stretched muscles of the pelvic floor and improve their blood supply. You should aim at doing this last exercise three times each half hour while in hospital: whilst at first it is easier lying maybe in the bath in the next six weeks it can be performed standing. Indeed, even after this time, the pelvic floor muscles will benefit if you do this daily for a long period.

Later

The following exercises may be added when advised.

Knee swinging

Lie on your back with your arms spread sideways, both knees bent and pressed together with feet on the bed. Correct the pelvic tilt as mentioned above, move both your knees first to one side and then to the other, making them touch the bed on either side with each movement. Keep your abdomen flat and firm.

For a low abdominal bulge

Lie flat with one knee bent on to the chest and the foot off the bed. Cross your arms in front, keep your chin in and raise both your head and the straight leg three inches off the bed. Lower both and relax. Repeat five times for each leg.

POST-NATAL CARE

For the sides of the waist

Lie on one side wi h the underneath knee bent to steady the position. Straighten the upper leg and raise it high. Repeat this five times; turn over and do the same on the other side.

Leg stretching

Lie with your legs straight and slide one leg down the bed as far as you can stretch it while at the same time drawing the knee of the other up to the waist so that it is as short as you can get it. Stretch each leg alternately keeping the pelvis corrected throughout the exercise.

Head raising

Lie on your back with both knees bent. Correct the pelvic tilt as described above and then draw in your chin and raise the head off the pillow. When able to do this without losing control of the pelvic correction, stretch your right hand towards the left knee and repeat to alternate sides.

Posture

Stand with your feet parallel and slightly apart. Straighten the knees and take the weight of the body on the balls of the feet. Correct the pelvic tilt by drawing in the abdomen and tightening the bottom muscles. Raise the ribs, lengthen the back of the neck and try to 'grow taller'. Breathe easily and walk freely in the corrected position.

Try to set aside a certain time every day for your exercises followed by complete relaxation to rest the whole body. It is often easier to find two periods of a quarter of an hour than a full half hour. The best times are before going to bed at night and after the afternoon rest. Try to maintain a good posture, whether walking, standing or sitting, even while doing the housework, and take a brief walk every day in the fresh air practising deep breathing.

Post-natal Examination

When a woman is delivered in a hospital, she is examined before she goes home. This will include an examination of the abdomen, breasts and legs. The uterus is felt through the abdominal wall and the entrance to the vagina inspected. The blood pressure is also usually recorded. This is a good time to ask the doctor any questions about points which are worrying you.

The second post-natal examination takes place between the fourth and sixth week after delivery; it includes an abdominal and pelvic examination as well as inspection of the cervix with a speculum. Many hospitals use this opportunity to take a cervical smear. This is a painless test whereby the surface cells of the cervix are removed by gentle rubbing and transferred to a glass slide for microscopic examination. It is a valuable health procedure for women and should be done anyway every few years in a woman's reproductive life. This public health measure is often combined with the post-natal examination for convenience of the mother.

At this second examination the breasts are usually examined, the urine tested, and blood pressure and weight recorded. It is sad that about a third of women do not make use of the services provided at such an examination. Whilst the emphasis in this country is still on ante-natal examination and care, it is important to have an additional examination some weeks after delivery so as to try to forestall any complications which could arise at a later date. Many minor problems can be prevented by proper post-natal examinations: vaginal discharge can be treated at this time, backache alleviated, bladder trouble corrected and lax muscles treated by physiotherapy. The cervix may have an erosion or ulcer which is a common cause of discharge. All these are potentially curable.

There are other important things to be considered at the time of the post-natal examination; this is the time when the mother should establish her future contraceptive policy. It is important that a child's arrival in a family is when the parents wish it, and family planning is an integral part of post-natal examination. Occasionally this is actually done at the same clinic, sometimes it is done at a different clinic run by an outside agency, such as the Family Planning Association, or by the Area Health Authorities. Apart from enabling people to have babies when they want them, family planning gives mothers the necessary rest that their health requires between the birth of each child and allows both husband and wife to have and enjoy sexual intercourse without the fear of pregnancy.

There are many methods of contraception in common use these days. The oral contraceptive pill is becoming one of the more popular in many areas of this country in the age group of women currently attending maternity units. It is easy to take and once the woman is on a regular cycle she can forget her fears about pregnancy. Some women have been worried by exaggerated reports of major complications. These are very rare and produce a much smaller risk to life than the risk of the pregnancy which might have occurred had contraception not been used. Most of these risks were common when a high dose of oestrogen in the pill was in use. There are now low-dose oral contraceptives which are much safer. In addition to the serious side effects of the high-dose oestrogen pill, there can be some lesser complications which may well require you to take advice from your doctor.

The intra-uterine device or coil is another popular method used widely. Here a small plastic coil is slipped inside the uterus and prevents any pregnancies from occurring. Insertion is a painless procedure and the coil can be removed when further pregnancies are desired. Again, there is a small minor complication rate and you are best advised to consult your doctor as to whether such a form of contraception is suitable for you.

The older methods of a diaphragm inside the vagina or a sheath worn over the penis are both still widely used and have the great advantages of being cheap and easy to use. However, they do have failure rates and they may diminish some sensation in either partner at the time of intercourse. The use of contraceptive chemical foams and pessaries placed in the vagina is becoming less popular as their unreliability is being more widely realized.

There are now many doctors who are experts in this field of family planning. The mother would do well to take their advice, for they can help her choose the method which is best for her own situation. It is at the second post-natal examination that the chain of events leading to proper contraception should start, for it is here that the mother is considered to have finally wound up the pregnancy.

Another aspect of the post-natal examination is that it provides an opportunity for examination of the child. The baby may well have attended infant welfare clinics with his mother. If he has not, he should certainly be seen at the time the mother attends for post-natal examination. He should be examined, weighed and inquiries made about feeding habits. Now is the time also to start planning the immunization programme against disease which will go on for some years in his early life. Usually an infant welfare clinic is housed close to the post-natal clinic and so both examinations can take place at the same time, saving the mother the bother of going to two different clinics. If this is not so, a paediatrician is often in attendance at the post-natal clinic.

Should the mother be attending her family doctor for her post-natal examination, he can give advice about the baby at the same time.

Post-natal care is a good example of preventive medicine. Prevention is better than cure and at a post-natal examination abnormalities can be easily detected and put right at an early stage. Discuss any minor ailments: you can be reassured if there is nothing to worry about, or treated if there is. Many women unfortunately still believe that the price they have to pay for bringing children into the world is ill health. Much of this is unnecessary and can be prevented. In addition, a programme of proper contraception and of good infant care can be started at the time of the post-natal examination so that both mother and baby can be assured of their future health.

Chapter 8

BABY CARE AND FEEDING

THE first excitement about the new baby soon passes and the mother will find herself fully occupied in watching and interpreting his reactions. She may feel that she wants to keep him by her side all the time to get to know him more quickly. In the hospital environment the baby is often moved to the nursery for certain periods of the day and often at night time as well. This is one of the minor disadvantages of hospitals, but is essential to give the mother some rest: one fractious child can keep six mothers awake, only one of whom is directly concerned with that baby.

The mother who has just had her first baby should take every opportunity to learn about the management of her baby's feeding and hygiene while in the hospital. The midwives there will be able to help her with matters of bathing, clothing and changing nappies. She will then be able to return home feeling less apprehensive about handling her baby on her own. The first night after leaving the hospital can be an anxious one and mothers get worried about this. If you have had a home delivery your midwife will be visiting you every day for ten days or so. After this she may well be required in some local authority areas to visit, at less frequent intervals, up to twenty-eight days. Anyway, she or the health visitor who takes over from her, will be of help to you in the home whether your baby was born there or whether you have just returned from hospital. Such skilled help can be most reassuring. They will help you care for the baby and with any problems you may have with his feeding, and will also check that he is developing normally. Infant welfare clinics are now available in all parts of the country and your health visitor will help you get an appointment at one. If you are still worried you may decide to talk to your family doctor or take your baby to see him.

The vast majority of babies develop perfectly normally and have no problems but this is little consolation to the mother who has never had one before. The smallest red spot may appear to be more serious when it is first seen than it does in the light of subsequent reflection, and the reassurance of someone who has handled many babies is most helpful and usually banishes worries. Should you have any serious problems, contact your health visitor or family doctor.

Infant Feeding

To many women the first basic question is whether to breast-feed the baby or not. A hundred years ago the subject was not discussed so much as it is today. In those days mothers never thought of feeding their babies other than with human milk. If for some reason the mother herself could not make enough milk then the wet-nurse was available. This was a woman who, having given birth to her own child, was still making milk and so could provide it for somebody else's baby. She was most helpful and was a true friend in times of need, but then there were not the well-established alternatives of artificial feeding which are available today.

There are still parts of the world where the arguments about breast-feeding are just not considered because mothers, grandmothers and great-grandmothers have always fed their babies naturally. This method of feeding is taken for granted and is as routine as any other bodily function. However, the world moves on and there are now excellent artificial feeds available for babies. The whole problem of breast-feeding is one charged with emotion and in this section we shall endeavour to try to separate the more scientific facts from the myths. There are really two questions to be answered: 'Is breast-feeding better for the baby?' and a second but equally important consideration, 'Is it more convenient?'

Undoubtedly for the human baby the correct feeding mixture in its early days is milk of its own species. The milk made in a mother's breasts contains the correct amount of foodstuffs in the right proportions – the baby's alimentary tract will very rarely be upset by his own mother's breast milk. This milk also contains a supply of the antibodies which help the body to fight against infection and these can cover the baby for the first few weeks of life when his own antibody production is very poor. In some parts of the world infective diarrhoea is a serious cause of illness and even death of children. In such places the breast-fed baby has an advantage over the artificially fed one for he is much more resistant to the effects of diarrhoea. This last argument is perhaps not a major one in this country but certainly applies in any semi-tropical climate where standards of hygiene are not very high. Thus, from the point of view of safety, there are many good arguments for breast-feeding.

Well-established breast-feeding probably also gains on the point of easiness and convenience. The equipment is always available and the milk is pre-sterilized ready for use. Little, therefore, has to be done in preparation for the feed. It should be stressed, however, that a breast-fed baby can only be fed by one person – the mother herself – and so on the score of ease artificial feeding may benefit, for more than one person can look after the child. If the mother should be ill or tired, a relative or friend can bottle-feed the baby just as easily as the mother, but nobody can substitute for her in breast-feeding.

An argument sometimes considered against breast-feeding

is that it may affect the shape of the breasts for subsequent years. This is probably untrue for it is the pregnancy and its incidental hormone changes that may make a breast more droopy after a baby has been born – lactation and feeding maintained for some months probably produces less structural change than the pregnancy itself.

Some babies are born prematurely and the care of such infants is a skilled nursing matter. Their feeding, however, very much concerns the mother. Breast milk here is undoubtedly the best food even if it has to be diluted with water at first. Obviously in the early days a very small baby cannot be put to the breast for he will not suckle, but the expressed milk of the mother can be given by a bottle with a spinal teat or even by dripping it through a tube to the baby. In these cases the means of giving the feed are not important: the main thing is that the baby is getting human breast milk. Should the baby have to stay in a premature baby unit, the hospital usually provides facilities for the mother to stay in or close to that unit too so that she can continue to supply milk for her baby.

There is less heat in the arguments for and against breast-feeding in the 1970s. If the woman wishes to and if it is easy to get well established, breast-feeding is a good method of feeding a baby. Should it not work easily, then artificial feeding is an excellent substitute. About a quarter of the women in this country breast-feed their child up to six weeks and the other three-quarters make use of the many alternatives available on the market.

So much for the meal itself, but there is also a psychological side to breast-feeding, i.e. its effect on the relationship between mother and baby. In the first few months of the baby's life a bond develops between them and this union helps the baby to gain a confidence which will be of great value in the future. A baby needs to be fondled and a breast-fed child seems to get more intimate contact with his mother than a bottle-fed one. It would certainly be difficult to hold a child to the breast four or five times a day for half an hour without a bond springing up between that child and its mother. A bottle-fed baby can also establish an equally strong psychological association with his mother if he is fondled in a similar way at the time of feeding, the important factor being not the type of feed but the attitude of the person feeding.

This does not mean that breast-feeding, being a natural and spontaneous process, needs no effort or preparation. A certain amount of teaching is needed; it is in the beginning that effort is particularly necessary for once a mother is familiar with this strange experience all will be well. It does mean taking a certain amount of trouble and the mother must strike a balance between taking enough and taking too much. Attitude of mind is important and will play a part in making a success of breast-feeding. A tense mind starts making difficulties before they occur and a vicious circle develops. There is no doubt that the placid mother usually finds her lactation period an easy one. Feeding should be attempted in a relaxed state of mind and body. In order to prevent backache the correct position for nursing should be used: the back must be firmly supported in a chair, the feet raised on a low stool and the holding arm resting on some support (not normally provided by the nursing chair, which has no arms).

Attention must be paid to preparation of the breasts for feeding. This should start in early pregnancy when the breasts should be examined by the doctor or midwife. If this examination is left until later it may be difficult to get any problems corrected in time. When the nipples are flat, the baby may not be able to grip on and suck properly. The wearing of special glass shells, designed by the late Dr Harold

BABY CARE AND FEEDING

Waller of the British Hospital for Mothers and Babies at Woolwich, can help to evert them. These shields can be worn under the brassiere for a good many weeks during pregnancy after which time the nipples will probably be more protuberant.

Towards the end of pregnancy a secretion (colostrum) develops in the breasts. It is rather like watered-down milk; some women like to express or squeeze out this fluid with the hand so as to establish an easy flow and prepare for the full flow of milk after the birth of the baby. Breast expression is difficult to learn on your own – you will be shown how to do it by your doctor or midwife.

Some mothers get worried about changes in the appearance of the milk itself in the first few days after delivery. These changes are quite normal; colostrum is usually expressed for a day or two after the birth. There is not a great deal of this, and so the baby should not be allowed to stay too long at the breast at this time when learning to suckle. On the third or fourth day the breasts usually get fuller and the milk becomes more plentiful and yellow. Then, over the space of a week, the full milk, which has a bluish colour, is to be seen. As the milk supply becomes more established, filling of the breasts will be noticed. The baby feeds more easily now and after a matter of only a few minutes he will become satisfied and fall asleep. He should not be put back in the cot right away, but a few minutes should be spent in helping him to bring up his wind. This is an instinctive movement which you can pick up from relations who have had babies or from your midwife or health visitor. The movement is a mixture of rubbing and patting the baby's back when he is in an upright position. It is not a boxing match so do not thump him but only pat.

Most children lose a few ounces in weight during the first week however they are fed, and they usually make up their birth weight after ten days or so. There is no need to be anxious about the baby's loss of weight in these early days but if you are worried ask your doctor or midwife: they can examine the baby to ensure normality and correctness of feeding methods.

It is not a good thing for the mother to have her relations in the room in the first few days when she is feeding the baby, especially if she is trying breast-feeding for the first time. She needs to be free from distractions at this time and a certain concentration is necessary even when breast-feeding has been established for some weeks. Once properly established, the whole procedure is very easy and does not demand concentration. Many women can talk to others or even read a book while still carrying on feeding their child. Others prefer not to do this but to concentrate entirely on the infant. You should do whichever comes naturally.

There is no need to keep your baby to a rigid time-table. The best tendency is to put him to the breast when he seems to be hungry – whatever the time may be. Mothers soon learn to recognize the cry and restlessness of hunger, especially late at night. No good can possibly be gained by allowing a baby to cry because he is hungry and keeping the whole house awake. Sometimes the very opposite may happen and the baby may sleep on past his regular feeding time. There is no harm in letting him do this for he will soon let you know when he is hungry.

You may be prescribed some medicines or even take some from the medicine cabinet from a previously prescribed bottle. It is as well to be aware that breast-fed infants may be affected by some of the drugs that the mother has taken. Laxatives such as senna, cascara or aloes may cause diarrhoea or colic in babies. Excessive consumption of alcohol or nicotine through cigarette smoking may also affect the baby. Barbiturates in sleeping tablets also pass into the milk; since they are amongst the most popular sedatives, caution is required in the amount that is taken.

For various reasons breast-feeding may not be the right method for you and you will then be advised about artificial feeding. Further, many mothers do not wish to breast-feed and their wishes are to be respected. One of the advances of recent times is the production of dried milks which are easier to prepare and safer for babies than liquid cow's milk. It is important that the bottle and teat are sterilized carefully to avoid infection. You will be advised about the amounts of feed and times by your midwife and health visitor. When in doubt, follow their directions exactly.

Generally speaking the proprietary milk feeds come in two strengths. Whilst many babies can go on to 'full strength' from the beginning, some require a few days on the 'half strength' mix first. Take the advice of your own midwife or health visitor about this. Of the various brands, all the reputable firms make a safe, proper milk mixture but different brands suit different babies. Start with the brand recommended and used most in the hospital you attend or by the health visitor you see. Your advisers will know that particular feed best and will therefore be able to help you assess whether it suits the baby. If it does not, take their advice as to which other milk you should use.

It is hard to overfeed a new baby (they regurgitate excess) but it can be done. Feed according to weight requirements rather than age and follow the instructions on the side of the can or packet exactly, making sure to use the correct proportion of water to powdered milk. When preparing a meal, the best dishes are made by following the recipe exactly: it is the same with making up bottle feeds.

Some mothers are bitterly disappointed when they fail to breast-feed and develop a guilt feeling. This is quite wrong, since the failure may be due to something over which they have no control. At present in this country three-quarters of the babies are bottle-fed. They do not seem any the worse for the experience. The important thing is to develop a method of feeding which is acceptable to you and the baby and then to persevere with it. The best infant feeding is that which suits both the baby and the mother.

Chapter 9

PROBLEMS IN PREGNANCY

MOST women go through pregnancy and have their baby with no major complications. However, sometimes problems do arise and their doctors and midwives have to advise treatments about which the mother may wonder. She may be surprised that her advisers are making her take certain courses of action when she is apparently feeling so healthy. It is not our intention to write a mini text-book of medicine in this volume but mothers have suggested to the authors that it might be useful if some of these conditions were mentioned so that if they arise in pregnancy you will understand why your advisers decided to take this particular course of action.

Pre-eclampsia. This is a condition in later pregnancy when the blood pressure is raised and the body becomes puffy because of retention of water. It is often associated with an alteration of the function of the placenta – the exchange station between the baby and mother. In its mildest form there is puffiness of the ankles and hands with a slight rise of blood pressure; this will have been detected in the ante-natal clinic. Later the blood pressure may rise even more and the kidneys become less efficient as filters so that protein appears in the urine. In its early stages pre-eclampsia can be treated with increased rest at home and some restriction of activity. If the condition worsens, however, many doctors will admit the mother to hospital to have increased bed rest. It is easier to rest in a hospital for up to twenty-four hours a day if somebody else is doing the everyday tasks and chores, cooking and making the beds for example. Should the condition require admission to hospital, sedative drugs are often given to help the mother rest and help lower the blood pressure. The other important feature of bed rest is that it increases the flow of blood to the placenta and so improves the supply of oxygen and foodstuffs to the unborn child.

In pre-eclampsia the fetus is often being supplied by a placenta that is not one hundred per cent efficient and sometimes it is felt that the baby should be delivered before the due date and so labour is started early by the doctor (see p. 77). All this sounds very formidable but provided the mother has been to the ante-natal clinic and her blood pressure has been checked regularly her advisers will be aware of any problems. Pre-eclampsia is not the dangerous condition it was thirty years ago and with modern regimens most women come through this condition and are returned to full health with a normal baby. The mother can best make sure of this happening if she follows her doctor's advice and rests when he tells her.

Bleeding in early pregnancy. If the egg is fertilized it settles into the lining of the womb within a few days. From then on most women do not bleed at all until after delivery and so there are no menstrual periods. If any bleeding from the vagina should occur, the doctor ought to be informed immediately. He will then take appropriate action to help you and your baby.

In the first three months of pregnancy this symptom may be associated with a threat that the uterus is trying to expel the fetus. Sometimes the uterus becomes more active and the baby is in jeopardy of being miscarried. The best treatment for this is to rest in bed completely until a day or so after the fresh bleeding has stopped. Such a situation is not irrevocable in its early stages and can be helped by following the doctor's advice and resting.

PROBLEMS IN PREGNANCY

A very small number of women are shown to be deficient in the hormone progesterone. If this is so the doctor can correct it by giving the hormone to the mother, thus maintaining the pregnancy. Another small group of women may have some weakness at the cervix – the neck of the uterus. These women have usually had previous deliveries or miscarriages or maybe had surgery such as dilation performed on the cervix. Such a group may benefit from a small operation which will tighten up the cervix. This is done under anaesthetic and usually means spending a few days in hospital, but it is well worth it if the pregnancy can be maintained.

In a few cases, the bleeding which may appear in early pregnancy will not come from the uterus itself but from lower down on the cervix or even the vagina. It may be caused by the presence of small ulcers or an infection of the vagina. Your doctor will be able to determine this by a simple examination with a small speculum which allows him to see the lining of the vagina and the surface of the cervix. Treatments can be given for these conditions but very often a doctor's hand may be stayed because of pregnancy. Bleeding from these conditions is not usually prejudicial to the health of the unborn baby.

Bleeding from the vagina in late pregnancy. Often labour starts with a 'bloody show' and a little more blood may be lost in the early stages of labour. This is due to the cervix being pulled up and separating from the membranes which surround the baby. Except for this, there should be no bleeding in late pregnancy. Any that occurs should be reported to the doctor immediately. A common cause of this symptom is the low implantation of the placenta. When the egg is fertilized it settles in the uterus, usually in the upper part. Very occasionally, however, the fertilized egg implants in the lower part of the uterus. As it grows and the placenta is formed, the latter spreads over the lower part of the uterus so that part of it comes near to the internal opening of the uterus at the cervix. Thus, in later pregnancy, there may be a little bleeding; the blood passes through the cervix into the vagina and appears at the vulva. This condition could obviously be dangerous at the time of delivery and might indeed be a barrier to the baby's progress.

Tests using X-rays or Ultrasound can be carried out to detect the site of the placenta. Should it be low-lying it may be necessary for the baby to be born by a Caesarean section, for he cannot be delivered if the placenta is in the way. Unfortunately this condition sometimes appears when the mother still has six or eight weeks to go in her pregnancy. Whilst the diagnosis could be made fairly soon, it would obviously be unwise to deliver the baby then unless the doctor's hand is forced by excessive blood loss and this rarely happens. Such a baby delivered at thirty-two weeks would only weigh three or four pounds and would suffer from the problems of immaturity. It is the practice therefore in this country to try to maintain the pregnancy for a few weeks longer before delivering despite the knowledge that the placenta is low down. This is not hazardous provided the mother is under constant supervision, which means admission to hospital and staying there. Such treatment may sound an imposition, especially when there are other children in the family, but a little thought will show the mother that it is the best course not just for her but for her unborn child.

Another cause of bleeding in later pregnancy is the separation of the normally sited placenta from its bed in the uterus. This is a serious condition, often accompanied by pain and occasionally by premature labour. The mother should be taken to hospital and kept under the care of skilled personnel in order that the best chances of a good result for her and the baby are available. Again a Caesarean section and blood transfusion may be required, but these will be done at the discretion of the doctor in charge of the case.

The same kind of bleeding from local causes in the cervix and vagina may occur in late as in early pregnancy. Again these can be diagnosed and dealt with appropriately. They are not usually serious and do not affect the mother or baby permanently.

The Rhesus effect. Besides the well-known blood groups, A, B and O, human blood can be classified using another grouping system called the Rhesus factor. Eighty-five per cent of the population are Rhesus positive (Rh+) and fifteen per cent are Rhesus negative (Rh−). If a mother who is Rhesus negative marries a Rhesus-positive man, her baby may inherit a Rhesus-positive trend from the father. Should some of the red blood cells from a Rhesus-positive unborn child leak across the placenta into the mother they could stimulate the formation of Rhesus antibodies in the defensive tissues of the mother. These can then pass back across the placenta to the baby in the uterus and can destroy his red blood cells causing him to become anaemic or jaundiced, two serious complications. Whilst fetal red blood cells can leak across to the mother at any time in pregnancy, the most likely time for this to happen is during and just after delivery, particularly when the placenta is being delivered. This is obviously too late to affect the baby in the current pregnancy but it may be the cause of antibody troubles in future babies. After the primary sensitization of the mother's defensive mechanisms by the fetal blood cells, subsequent stimulation by even a few Rhesus-positive red blood cells causes a very brisk response and so later pregnancies might be affected while the child is still in the uterus.

Only about one person in seven is Rhesus negative. Thus by chance in only one in eight marriages is the mother Rh− and the father Rh+. The Rhesus factor causes trouble in only a small proportion of even these pregnancies with mixed Rhesus groups, harmful antibodies developing in fact only in about one in 200 pregnancies. The risk during the first pregnancy of a Rhesus-negative mother having her baby affected is negligible unless she has had a previous blood transfusion with Rhesus-positive blood. Even with her subsequent pregnancies, the background chance of her having a baby who is not affected by jaundice or anaemia is nine out of ten.

The whole management of the Rhesus problem has been helped by the discovery in the mid 1960s of an injection which can be given to the Rh− mother immediately after delivery. This prevents any of the baby's Rh+ red cells which may have crossed to the mother during childbirth from sensitizing her, so the mother does not make any of the offending Rhesus antibodies. Thus each subsequent pregnancy, from the immunological point of view, is as though she were having her first baby, i.e. a situation of low risk. The Rhesus problem will be overcome provided these injections are given correctly to all mothers in need of them.

It is usual in most hospitals dealing with this problem for the mother to have her blood checked when she comes to the ante-natal clinic in early pregnancy. Antibody levels are assessed at intervals throughout pregnancy, and a day or so after delivery, an injection of anti-Rhesus gamma globulin is given to the Rh− mother.

A few babies will obviously still be born whose mothers have been sensitized before the use of anti-Rhesus gamma globulin started. For these, new research also brings more hope. The state of the baby inside the uterus can be checked by the antibody tests of the mother's blood and by drawing off a little of the fluid surrounding the baby inside the uterus. This can be checked for blood breakdown products and should the baby be badly affected he can receive treatment by transfusion even while he is still in the uterus. Usually an affected baby will be delivered earlier and he will then receive further treatment by means of exchange transfusions. This last group of affected babies is getting smaller and within the next fifteen years will be even further reduced. However, should any baby escape the net of prevention of the anti-D gamma globulin he will be caught and treated by the curative treatment which has now been developed to a high degree of perfection in specialist maternity units.

The production of excess fluid. Before birth the baby lives in a sac surrounded by fluid. This is made partly by the membranes surrounding the baby and partly by the unborn child himself. It is his protection in later pregnancy, buffering him from the mechanical jolts of the outside world and providing an even temperature and an almost gravity-free existence in which to grow and move easily. Occasionally, however, too much fluid is made and this over-distends the uterus causing the mother to have stretch symptoms. These are painful and, on examination, the uterus will be found to be much bigger than normal for that time in pregnancy. Often this condition can be resolved by making the patient rest; the excess fluid is re-absorbed and the uterus returns to its normal size. Occasionally, however, if the patient is in severe pain some of the fluid may be drawn off through the mother's abdominal wall. This is not a painful procedure for a little local anaesthetic is injected first and the withdrawal should have no ill effect on the baby. Occasionally, however, the presence of excess fluid – *hydramnios* – is associated with some problem of the baby, such as the presence of twins, and doctors often will take an X-ray of a mother with this condition in order to exclude the possibility of these problems.

A much rarer problem is a lack of this amniotic fluid. In this case the baby can be felt very readily through the mother's abdominal wall and the containing uterus. This condition is not often diagnosed but may be associated with the onset of premature labour.

Urinary infection in pregnancy. The bladder and urinary tract are more susceptible to infection during pregnancy than at other times. The normal hormones of pregnancy may cause the bladder and tubes draining from the kidneys to be more flaccid and so some of the urine may stagnate in the urinary tract. Further, in late pregnancy the baby's head presses down the pelvis and this also may be a cause of retention of a small pool of urine. All this leads to the sort of condition which can give rise to infection and mothers would do well to drink plenty of fluid in pregnancy in order to try to keep the urinary fluids moving.

Mothers who have an infection of the urinary tract usually get a burning pain on passing water. This scalding sensation often appears at the beginning and end of the act of urinating. The symptom of increased frequency is not so significant in pregnancy because many women pass urine more often just because of the pressure of the growing uterus and baby. If, however, this increased desire to pass urine is accompanied by burning, medical advice should be sought. Often a special specimen of urine will be checked to see if there are any bacteria in it and treatment can be readily given. In order to aid this treatment a lot of fluid must be drunk to keep the urine flowing freely. Urinary infection will not be a serious condition in pregnancy provided it is treated early with proper chemotherapy and high fluid intake.

Anaemia. During pregnancy, the growing baby and his

placenta demand large amounts of iron from the mother. Even if the iron intake of the mother is poor, the baby will still get this iron, taking it from the maternal tissues, causing the mother to become anaemic. It is largely to try to prevent this problem that the mother is given supplies of iron in early pregnancy. This daily taking of iron tablets is an attempt not just to prevent anaemia but to build up iron stores in mother and baby. Usually a blood test is performed in early pregnancy and repeated once or twice later on. This gives the doctor a chance to make sure anaemia has not started and most women, if they take iron tablets throughout pregnancy, do not get this condition. Should it occur the doctor will treat it either by altering the form of iron being taken orally or possibly by giving iron injections which will by-pass the absorptive areas of the intestines thus ensuring that the iron gets into the system. Very rarely in this country do mothers become so anaemic that they require a blood transfusion towards the end of pregnancy. This is given when the doctor feels that there is not enough time left in the pregnancy for the mother to build up her own blood reserves before labour is likely to start. It would be dangerous for a mother to go into labour if she were anaemic and doctors usually try to overcome this problem before labour starts.

Abdominal pain in pregnancy. Many women get stretch pains as the uterus grows but a pain more serious than this should be reported to the doctor. Often there is no serious underlying condition but it is still advisable for him to determine this. Appendicitis can still occur in pregnant women as it can in the non-pregnant and it is better for your doctor to decide whether the pain is a serious one or not.

Other medical conditions. Not many years ago women who had chronic medical conditions, such as diabetes or heart disease, were not allowed to have children. This situation has altered and now such women can quite safely deliver normal babies provided they are medically supervised during pregnancy and delivery. If a woman has such a condition she would probably do well to talk to her doctor before thinking of having a baby but in most cases women who were previously considered to be unsuitable for pregnancy can now go ahead with perfect safety under the care of expert obstetricians. Obviously extra precautions will have to be taken and the mother may well have to spend some part of her pregnancy in hospital, but these are considered by many women a small price to pay for the satisfaction of producing their own children.

Chapter 10

SOME QUESTIONS MOTHERS ASK

At most ante-natal clinics meetings are arranged for the expectant mothers and their husbands to meet the doctors and the midwives responsible for maternity care. At these group meetings questions are encouraged and parents can discuss any anxieties. Many women prefer to ask their questions in the more private conditions of the ante-natal examination when they are alone with the doctor or midwife. Experience of both these situations has shown that lack of authentic knowledge plays an important part in making pregnancy an anxious time.

There are some constantly recurring questions and a few of these will be answered in this chapter. Perhaps there is no subject about which there are so many half-truths, so much superstition and, in consequence, fear, as having a baby. As an example of a longstanding superstition, a mother recently asked one of the authors at an ante-natal clinic, 'Do things you do before the baby is born affect him? I put my tongue out at my husband and my mother-in-law said that my baby would be born tongue-tied.' This is obviously nonsense but even intelligent people cannot differentiate in times of high emotion between nonsense and practical possibility. Recently we looked after an intelligent woman who had taken a good first-class degree at one of the older universities. She was tense and anxious throughout pregnancy and no amount of discussion could alleviate this. It was not until a week after her normal delivery that she explained the problem. She had read about Mary Tudor who was alleged to have had a twenty-month pregnancy.

Although this mother knew that most women gave birth after a nine-month pregnancy she secretly wondered if there could be exceptions and she was afraid that she, like Mary, was such an exception and might continue to be pregnant for almost two years. This was a misunderstanding that could have been easily corrected had she ever felt able to ask questions and to talk freely. There is no truth in the tale about Queen Mary; in fact, she was never pregnant. The problem seemed too silly for our patient to mention to any of us, and so it festered in her mind.

Questions Relating to Pregnancy

Why do some pregnancies end in abortion?

Spontaneous abortion or miscarriage is quite common, occurring in one in ten pregnancies. The cause is not known but sometimes there is a history of a fall, sudden exertion, or even a serious accident. The commonest cause is that there is an abnormality of the fertilized ovum and so the baby would never have developed properly. This is Nature's way of controlling the quality of the species.

The likeliest time for an abortion to occur is between the eighth and twelfth weeks of pregnancy. When a woman has had one or more abortions she naturally becomes anxious about ever being able to carry a pregnancy through. It is wise to seek gynaecological advice for proper investigations, treatment with hormones or surgery might help such a woman carry a full-term pregnancy.

Need I wear a special support or corset during pregnancy?

It is seldom necessary to wear a support unless your abdominal muscles are weak. It is good to exercise muscles during pregnancy and the days have fortunately gone when women trussed themselves up in bone corsets, being forbidden to take exercise or move about while carrying their baby. Occasionally, however, an elastic roll-on is helpful, especially for those used to it.

Does the pelvis expand during pregnancy?

Yes, it is natural for the joints of this part of the body to widen a little due to the influence of the hormone progesterone which softens the ligaments guarding these joints. Thus the capacity of the pelvis is enlarged and whilst making it easier for the passage of the fetal head, it does occasionally lead to some weakness in the big joints of the lower back which bear the weight of the body. If excessive work is done at this time of lax ligaments, permanent weakness could follow, giving rise to backache.

How long should I go on working?

It all depends on the kind of job you are doing. If it is not tiring work and you can sit down, it should be possible for you to go on until about six weeks before the expected date of birth. Towards the end of pregnancy it is important to give up some time each day for resting and you cannot do this in certain jobs. On the other hand, if the work involves standing then it should be stopped much earlier.

The financial status of the mother may be affected by her choice of when to stop work, for the Department of Health and Social Security will pay the maternity grant to anyone working up to thirteen weeks from the expected date of delivery; many women go on working until this time in order to qualify for the grant. Discussion with the medical social worker at the ante-natal clinic will help sort out this point.

Could a severe mental shock in early pregnancy affect the baby?

There is no scientific evidence of this. During the wars and civil disturbances of the last few years many expectant mothers have been caught in bombing and violent action; some have been severely injured, physically and emotionally. Despite these experiences miscarriages, premature births, birthmarks and deformities have not increased.

Can any infectious diseases of the mother affect the baby before birth?

There is proof that a mother who has had rubella or German measles during the first three months of pregnancy may have a baby affected by congenital disease – blindness, deafness or heart disease. During pregnancy, therefore, it is important to avoid contact with any person suffering from this. (The earlier in pregnancy that rubella is contracted, the higher the risk of any problem.) Should a pregnant woman either have this condition or have been in contact with German measles it is advisable for her to contact her doctor fairly quickly: he will give her advice and, if necessary, treatment. There is less evidence of other infections affecting the unborn child but any woman in early pregnancy would do well to keep clear of any person who has a known infection.

Is it possible to determine the sex of the baby during pregnancy?

This can be done by examination of the cells in the fluid surrounding the baby during pregnancy. However, this involves puncturing the abdomen and is not usually performed unless there is some good medical reason for determining the baby's sex. Beyond this method there is no reliable way of finding out what sex the unborn child is: the tests which involve apparatus like watches swung over the abdomen have no scientific truth behind them.

Why are some babies born prematurely?

In a number of cases premature birth is due to maternal disease, such as toxaemia of pregnancy or pre-eclampsia (see p. 77). In a great majority, however, the cause is unknown and much research is being concentrated on this subject. There is no reason why a baby born prematurely should not survive if he is given special care at birth and during the critical weeks which follow. He can grow up into an adult, normal both mentally and physically. Winston Churchill in later life showed no ill results of his premature birth; neither did Charles Darwin or Victor Hugo, both of whom were very small at birth.

If a mother has given birth to a baby with a congenital malformation what are the chances of this recurring in subsequent pregnancies?

The incidence of recurring congenital malformations varies enormously according to the type of abnormality. It is wise to take the advice of your obstetrician about the problem which is worrying you for he may be able to give you more exact advice in relation to that particular congenital malformation.

Is epilepsy hereditary?

There does seem to be a hereditary factor. Samples drawn from the general population show that about two and a half per cent of children with an epileptic parent are similarly affected. This figure is about five times greater than the general incidence of the condition.

What is the earliest time that twins can be diagnosed? How do they originate?

Twins may be suspected when the uterus is larger than normal. This is not usually noticed until the middle of pregnancy; most twins are diagnosed at thirty to thirty-four weeks. The medical attendant may be able to feel two separate heads. An X-ray examination is the most certain way of making the diagnosis and is not dangerous in late pregnancy. If the hospital has the equipment, Ultrasound pictures can also be used to confirm the diagnosis.

There is a geographical variation in the frequency of twin births. For instance, in parts of Asia this is 1 in 120 pregnancies whereas in Europe it is 1 in 80. Twins may be the result of the fertilization of a single egg or of two separate eggs. In the former case identical twins result, in the latter fraternal. Identical twins are always of the same sex and closely resemble each other. Fraternal twins are four times more frequent than identical twins.

It is usual for twin deliveries to be premature and they should always take place in hospital. Many obstetricians advise mothers who are expecting twins to attend the hospital more frequently and sometimes insist that the mother has extra bed rest as an in-patient. This helps to put off premature labour and allows the twins to be larger at birth.

Does a change in food habits matter?

Many women experience an increase in appetite, especially in the first three months. Even with the presence of nausea or heartburn this can still happen. Other women develop unusual cravings or aversions. The craving for fruit, milk, spicy or savoury foods is well recognized. Aversions to tea, coffee, eggs, fried food and smoking are quite common. These habits cause no ill effect to the unborn baby and, provided the cravings are indulged in moderation only, they do not affect the mother.

Why is it so important to restrict food intake?

Diet is one of the most important aspects of pregnancy over which the woman has some control. With the natural increase in appetite there is a tendency to overeat and put on excessive weight. Women who become overweight may have an increased risk of developing toxaemia which may lead to prematurity. This is not a very great risk but they will certainly remain overweight after the baby is born and with each successive pregnancy put on still more weight. It is far easier to prevent weight gain during pregnancy than it is to try to lose weight when there is a new baby in the house. Many women start on the downward path of increased weight with their pregnancies and it must be remembered that obesity is a serious disease in the mid forties for it is often associated with heart disease, high blood pressure, and diabetes.

What about immunization and the pregnant traveller?

The International Health Regulations adopted in May 1951 by most countries ensure maximum security against the major quarantinable diseases. When undertaking an international journey a pregnant woman should ask her doctor and travel agents about the mandatory immunization requirements for the particular country she is visiting. The commonest is immunization against smallpox.

Are smallpox vaccinations inadvisable on medical grounds because of pregnancy?

In brief, this is a question of assessing the risk of vaccination to the mother and her unborn child compared to that of contracting smallpox in endemic or infected areas. If a doctor genuinely feels that vaccination is inadvisable in pregnancy he should give the mother a certificate giving full details of the pregnancy. The airline or ship may permit travel in such cases but it must be appreciated that it is the Health Authority at the port of arrival which has the final decision on those arriving without valid certificates and passengers may be liable to inconvenience, delay, and even quarantine, at their final destination. Australia, for example, will rarely, if ever, accept medical certificates stating that vaccination against smallpox is contraindicated and an unvaccinated passenger will be liable to quarantine at the first port of call in Australia however compelling the clinical contraindications and whatever her doctor's certificate may say.

How late in pregnancy is it safe to fly?

As can be imagined, an aircraft is the last place one would choose to have a baby. Because of this and the possible risk of premature labour being induced by the physiological or psychological stresses of a long flight, pregnant women are not accepted on international journeys after the end of the thirty-fifth week of pregnancy. This may be extended slightly to the thirty-sixth week for domestic journeys. It is wise to check with the airline concerned, and if you are close to these times, get a certificate from the ante-natal clinic clearly giving the stage of pregnancy reached.

Questions Relating to Labour

Do pain-relieving drugs make labour last longer, or harm the baby? Does the use of gas and oxygen make labour longer?

Pain relief in labour – obstetric analgesia – is a subject about which much research is being done. Modern drugs, given properly, are not harmful. Neither gas and oxygen nor trilene make labour longer. The same can be said for pethidine. You are not compelled to have any pain relief but it is quite normal and harmless for you to do so.

Is it true that older women have a worse time with their first babies than younger women?

It depends what is meant by old. After the age of thirty a woman's fertility starts to decline. If she does conceive there is no reason at all why, with modern care and attention, she should be any worse off than her younger sisters.

Why do some women have to have an operative delivery?

There are many reasons – most of them quite beyond the control of the mother or the person looking after her. The commonest cause is that the uterus has become unable to complete the final delivery – usually on account of fatigue. When forceps are used, either a local or a general anaesthetic is given: this is completely painless. Other causes relate to the baby when the obstetrician feels that it is safer to deliver the baby soon rather than await any more delay, or that the baby is at a disadvantageous angle of approach for delivery.

Is it usual to have a haemorrhage at delivery?

A show of blood is a sign of the start of labour and this should not be considered to be a haemorrhage. With the delivery of the afterbirth (placenta) after the birth of the baby there is often some bleeding. This is controlled by your doctor or midwife who will have given an injection to help the uterus contract, allowing the normal loss of a few ounces only – the body can stand this. Should blood loss be more, your doctor can take action to stop this and so prevent serious complications.

Should my baby be circumcised?

There are very few medical reasons for so treating a baby. The foreskin of his penis is not intended to retract for two or three years and attempts to do so in the new born are resisted. However, if parents are keen to have this operation performed on their sons, it is wise to do it early (in the first week of life) for it upsets the baby far less then than a circumcision done when he is a year or so old.

These are only a few of the questions that are often asked. But you should not hesitate at all times to ask your doctor or midwife about anything that you want to discuss or have explained.

GLOSSARY

OFTEN doctors and midwives use technical terms when talking together and patients hear these. On other occasions such words may be used to the patient inadvertently by the doctor. He may leave the patient with some doubts as to the real meaning of what he is saying. In consequence, several patients have suggested that we give a list of words they may come across and whose meaning is not absolutely clear.

ABORTION: a pregnancy which finishes before twenty-eight weeks (seven months). The causes may be natural or not but the word covers both senses and does *not* only mean an induced abortion. It covers natural and spontaneous ones so that when a doctor uses the word he is not implying the same thing as many lay people do.

AMENORRHOEA: an absence of menstrual periods as happens in pregnancy.

ANALGESIA: the relief of pain by numbing the nerves or by dimming sensations. Usually in medicine this word does not include anaesthesia, which stops pain by making the patient completely unconscious.

AREOLA OF BREAST: the area of raised skin around the nipple which is pink before pregnancy but may turn brown later.

CATHETER: a thin hollow plastic or rubber tube used to release urine from the bladder if the patient is unable to void herself. Insertion is painless and the relief is great.

CERVIX: the entrance (and exit) of the uterus. A ring of muscle which dilates in labour from one to ten centimetres diameter to allow the baby to be born.

DIAPHRAGM: 1) a shelf of muscle across a body cavity such as the one in the pelvis which holds the uterus in place (see Eigure 16).

2) a rubber disk slipped into the vagina as a contraceptive to block the passage of sperm up into the uterus.

ECLAMPSIA: a condition of fits occurring in late pregnancy or labour. It is very rare now for proper ante-natal care can usually detect the early stages of this disease and good treatment can prevent it.

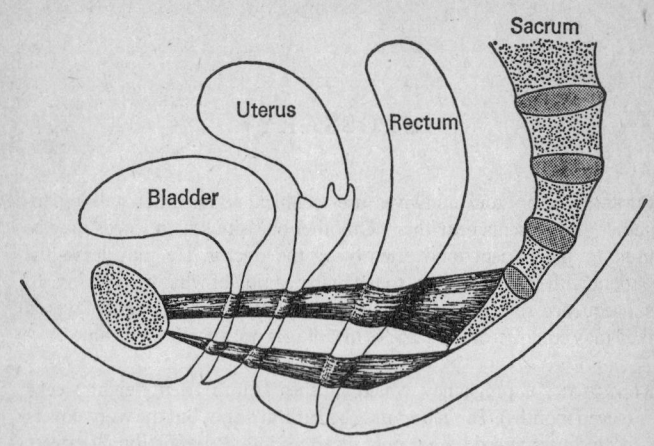

Figure 16 The muscles that make up the pelvic diaphragm.

EMBRYO: a baby in its earliest stages of development. The word is usually applied before about twelve weeks.

ENGAGEMENT: The passage of the widest diameter of the baby's head through the brim of the mother's pelvis. This often happens in the last few weeks of pregnancy and is a good sign of the probability of the baby being able to negotiate the whole pelvis.

EPISIOTOMY: a clean incision made in the perineum to ease the passage of the baby's head. It is usually done under local anaesthesia and heals far better than a ragged tear.

EROSION: an area of heaping up of cells on the surface of the cervix which may be associated with a vaginal discharge. It is not a cancer or even a pre-cancer and can be easily treated if it persists when pregnancy is over.

EXPRESSION (OF THE BREASTS): should the breasts be overfilled with milk after delivery, it is often necessary to remove it. This can be done by gentle hand massage or a small breast pump which puts an intermittent suction on the breast. Either of these methods expresses excess milk and leaves the breast less tense to continue further production of milk. Occasionally a baby is too small to be put to the breast. His mother's milk is still the best food and in this situation expressed breast milk can be used.

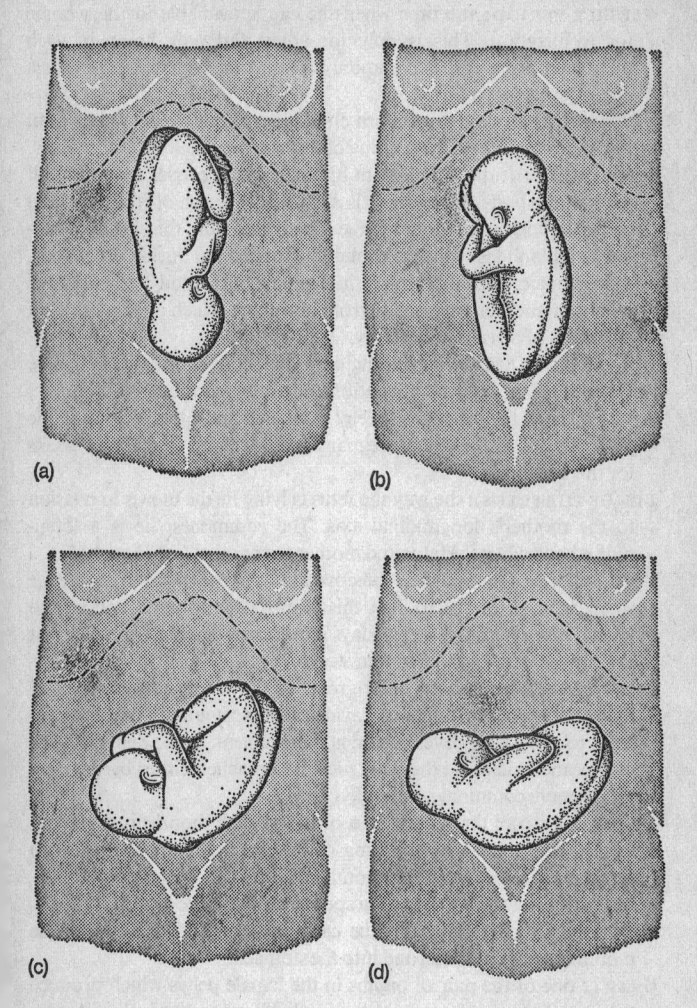

Figure 17 Lie of the fetus. Most common is a longitudinal lie, either head down (a) or buttocks down (b); less common are oblique (c) or transverse lies (d).

FERTILE PERIOD: the time when the egg is available in the woman for fertilization. This is only for about thirty-six hours in each menstrual cycle and is commonly around the fourteenth day of a 28-day cycle (see p. 27).

FETUS (OR FOETUS): the unborn child from about twelve weeks until birth. (For a note on the spelling of this word see p. 30.)

HAEMOGLOBIN: the red pigment in blood which carries oxygen to all parts of the body. When there is a chronic shortage of iron, the level of circulating haemoglobin in the blood drops and this can be detected by a blood test which is commonly carried out during pregnancy.

HORMONE: a chemical produced in one part of the body which affects organs in another part, e.g. thyroid hormones which affect the speed of growth of all cells in the body.

INHALATION: taking something into the body through the lungs. Gases enter the body by inhalation and are expelled by exhalation.

INVOLUTION: the process whereby the uterus and other organs in the pelvis return to their non-pregnant state. It takes four to six weeks for this to happen.

LIE (OF THE FETUS): the way the fetus is lying in the uterus in relation to the mother's longitudinal axis. The commonest lie is a longitudinal one when the fetus and mother are parallel (see Figure 17).

LOCHIA: after delivery, the protective lining of the uterus is shed over the next week or so. At first this is mixed with blood and so the lochial loss is red. Over a few days it decreases and fades in colour; it usually ceases after three to four weeks.

MEMBRANES: the unborn child grows in the uterus inside a bag of fluid. This protects him and provides an almost gravity-free environment to allow easy development and movement. To be delivered, the membranes enclosing the baby must be broached either by the doctor or, more commonly, naturally.

MENSTRUATION: the regular loss of blood each month in the adult female. It signifies the shedding of the uterine lining and that no pregnancy has occurred that month.

MISCARRIAGE: the lay term for a spontaneous abortion.

OESOPHAGUS: the gullet or tube carrying food and drink from the mouth through the chest and into the stomach.

OVARY: one of the pair of organs in the female pelvis which produce the eggs. They are about an inch and a half long and an inch wide.

OVUM: the egg developed in the ovary. In most women one ovum is ripened each month and is ready for fertilization in mid cycle.

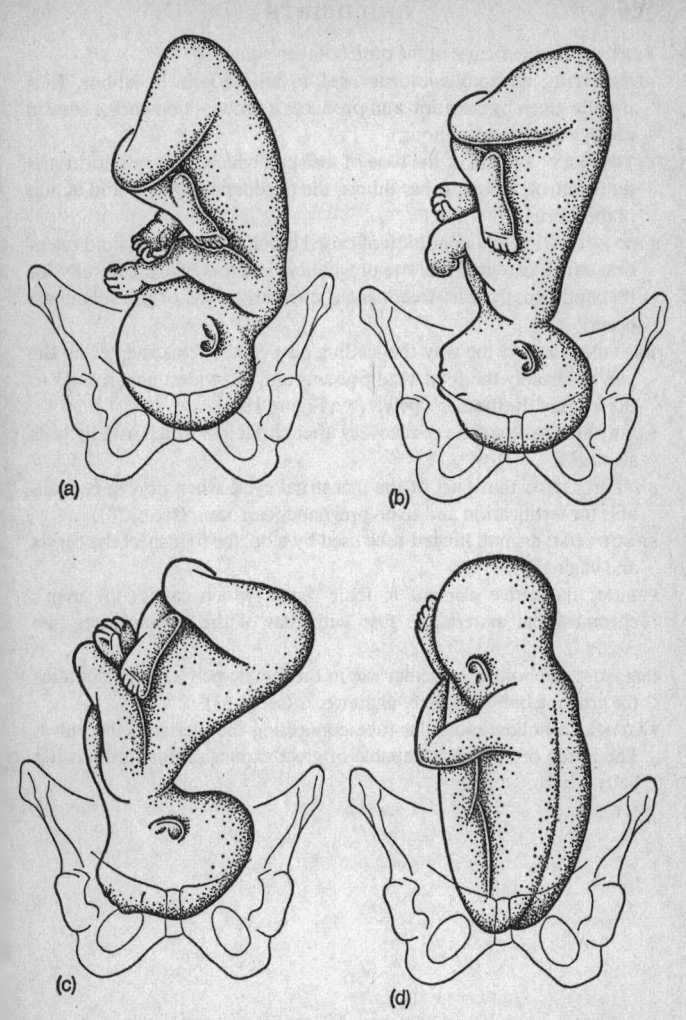

Figure 18 Presentation of the fetus. The most common presentation is by the head (cephalic), the chin well tucked down to the chest (a). Less common presenting parts are the brow (b) or the face (c). The buttocks present in 1 in 30 deliveries. This is a breech presentation (d).

PERINEUM: the tissues at the outlet of the vagina.

PETHIDINE: an analgesic drug used to relieve pain in labour. It is usually given by injection and produces a drowsy, non-caring state in about a quarter of an hour.

PITUITARY: a gland at the base of the skull which produces hormones that control, among other things, the production of eggs and action of the uterus.

PRE-ECLAMPSIA: a condition of raised blood pressure and fluid retention which can occur in late pregnancy. Doctors watch carefully for this and usually start treatment if any early signs of pre-eclampsia occur.

PRESENTATION: the way the leading part of the fetus is entering the pelvis. Usually the fetal head presents and the widest part rotates to the front of the mother's pelvis (see Figure 18).

PUERPERIUM: the time of recovery after childbirth which usually lasts six weeks.

SAFE PERIOD: that part of the menstrual cycle when no egg is available for fertilization and so no pregnancy can occur (see p. 28).

SPECULUM: a small hinged tube used by a doctor to inspect the cervix and vagina.

SPERM: the active element in male semen which carries the man's chromosomal material to fuse with that of the woman's egg (see p. 28).

UTERUS: the hollow muscular sac in the female pelvis which contains the growing baby for thirty-eight weeks (see p. 33).

VAGINA: a hollow muscular tube connecting the uterus to the vulva. The inside of its wall is capable of great expansion for through it a baby is born.

MORE ABOUT PENGUINS
AND PELICANS

Penguinews, which appears every month, contains details of all the new books issued by Penguins as they are published. From time to time it is supplemented by *Penguins in Print*, which is a complete list of all titles available. (There are some five thousand of these.)

A specimen copy of *Penguinews* will be sent to you free on request. For a year's issues (including the complete lists) please send 50p if you live in the British Isles, or 75p if you live elsewhere. Just write to Dept EP, Penguin Books Ltd, Harmondsworth, Middlesex, enclosing a cheque or postal order, and your name will be added to the mailing list.

In the U.S.A.: For a complete list of books available from Penguin in the United States write to Dept CS, Penguin Books Inc., 7110 Ambassador Road, Baltimore, Maryland 21207.

In Canada: For a complete list of books available from Penguin in Canada write to Penguin Books Canada Ltd, 41 Steelcase Road West, Markham, Ontario.

Dict P.52